W9-AUL-129

An Introduction to

Complementary and Alternative Therapies

Edited by
Georgia M. Decker, MS, RN,
CS-ANP, AOCN

Oncology Nursing Press, Inc.
A subsidiary of the Oncology Nursing Society
Pittsburgh, PA

Oncology Nursing Press, Inc.
Technical Publications Editor: Barbara Sigler, RN, MNEd
Staff Editor: Lisa M. George, BA
Creative Services Assistants: Chad Chronick, Dany Sjoen

An Introduction to Complementary and Alternative Therapies

Copyright © 1999 by the Oncology Nursing Press, Inc.

All rights reserved. No part of the material protected by this copyright may be reproduced or utilized in any form, electronic or mechanical, including photocopying, recording, or by an information storage and retrieval system, without written permission from the copyright owner. For information, write to the Oncology Nursing Press, Inc., 501 Holiday Drive, Pittsburgh, PA 15220-2749.

Library of Congress Card Catalog Number: 99-068395

ISBN 1-890504-14-9

Publisher's Note
This manual is published by the Oncology Nursing Press, Inc. (ONP). ONP neither represents nor guarantees that the practices described herein will, if followed, ensure safe and effective patient care. The recommendations contained in this manual reflect ONP's judgment regarding the state of general knowledge and practice in the field as of the date of publication. The recommendations may not be appropriate for use in all circumstances. Those who use this manual should make their own determinations regarding specific safe and appropriate patient-care practices, taking into account the personnel, equipment, and practices available at the hospital or other facility at which they are located. The editor and publisher cannot be held responsible for any liability incurred as a consequence from the use or application of any of the contents of these guidelines. Figures and tables are used as examples only. They are not meant to be all-inclusive, nor do they represent endorsement of any particular institution by the Oncology Nursing Society (ONS). Mention of specific products and opinions related to those products do not indicate or imply endorsement by ONS or ONP.

ONS and ONP publications are originally published in English. Permission has been granted by the ONS Board of Directors for foreign translation. (Individual tables and figures that are reprinted or adapted require additional permission from the original source.) However, because translations from English may not always be accurate and precise, ONS and ONP disclaim any responsibility for inaccurate translations. Readers relying on precise information should check the original English version.

Printed in the United States of America

Oncology Nursing Press, Inc.
A subsidiary of the Oncology Nursing Society

Dedication

To my patients, you are with me always. To my colleagues, it has been my honor to work with you. To my family and friends, without your understanding and support I could not have done this. All of you have provided inspiration and wisdom even when you did not always understand or agree with the importance of complementary therapies. Thank you.

Acknowledgments

I want to acknowledge the contributing authors who were willing to take the leap and think with an open mind. Your courage, knowledge, and tenacity made this book all I hoped it would be. Special thanks to Eleanor Milos for providing illustrations appearing in Chapters 2, 4, and 6 and to Jude Seney Melendez for her help with research, typing, editing, and the content in Chapter 4. The Oncology Nursing Press, Inc. provided a unique opportunity. Special thanks to Barbara Sigler and Lisa George.

Contributors

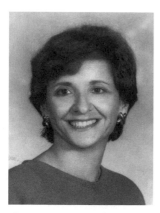

Georgia M. Decker, MS, RN, CS-ANP, AOCN
Founder and Advanced Practice Nurse, Integrative Care, Albany, NY

Chapter 2, Bioelectromagnetic Therapies; Chapter 4, Manual Healing Methods; Chapter 5, Pharmacologic and Biologic Therapies; Chapter 7, Diet, Nutrition, and Lifestyle Changes

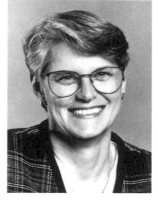

Linda U. Krebs, RN, PhD, AOCN
Assistant Professor, University of Colorado, School of Nursing, Denver, CO

Chapter 1, Mind-Body Interventions

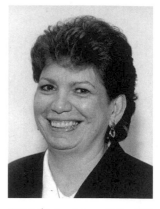

Wende L. Levy, RN, MS
Senior Clinical Trials Specialist, Social and Scientific Systems, Rockville, MD

Chapter 5, Pharmacologic and Biologic Therapies

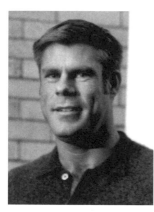

Michael Murray, RN, OCN®
Medical Consultant/Writer, Chicago, IL

Chapter 7, Diet, Nutrition, and Lifestyle Changes

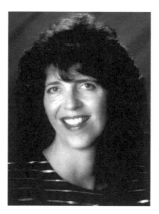

Jamie S. Myers, RN, MN, AOCN
Oncology Clinical Nurse Specialist, Research Medical Center, Kansas City, MO

Chapter 6, Herbal Medicine

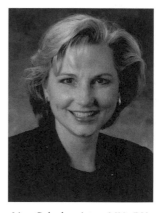

Lisa Schulmeister, MN, RN, CS, OCN®
Oncology Nursing Consultant, Member of the Stanley S. Scott Cancer Center, Adjunct Assistant Professor of Nursing, Louisiana State University Medical Center, New Orleans, LA

Chapter 3, Alternative Systems of Medical Practice

Table of Contents

Foreword

The imperative is clear: Whether providers agree or disagree with the use of complementary and alternative therapies, these interventions are an integral part of health care in the United States. In fact, today, the field of complementary and alternative therapies is growing 18 times faster than any other segment of health care (Porter-O'Grady, 1999). Forty-one percent of Americans surveyed by Eisenberg et al. (1998) used complementary and alternative therapies in 1997, up from 34% in 1990, at a conservatively estimated cost of $21.2 billion. At least $12.2 billion is paid out of pocket. Many people who use complementary and alternative therapies do not tell their healthcare providers, and until recently, doctors, nurses, social workers, and others received very little education about alternative and complementary therapies. Although the National Institutes of Health established the Office of Complementary and Alternative Medicine to help us learn more, healthcare providers still take a "don't ask, don't tell" approach. Clinical practice must change to respond to the healthcare needs of the U.S. population.

The challenge is to increase our own understanding about complementary and alternative therapies, remain open-minded and consider them as part of care management, and include questions about these therapies as a routine part of patient assessment and evaluation.

An Introduction to Complementary and Alternative Therapies can help. Finally, there's a user-friendly book that will help a vast audience to learn more about alternative and complementary therapies in health care! This book clearly meets the authors' goals of providing a quick and easy "hands-on" reference and list of resources that can be used as part of daily clinical practice. It should be required as a ready reference for all healthcare providers, yet it is written in a manner that makes the information accessible for the lay audience, as well. The book provides a comprehensive, yet brief and easy-to-read, description of many alternative and complementary therapies, with special considerations for each intervention. Also included is a comprehensive list of resources that can provide further information on many of the topics. Readers will learn about a variety of therapies, including mind-body interventions, pharmacologic and biologic therapies, herbal therapies, nutrition and lifestyle, alternative systems of medicine, and much more. Many of our patients are routinely using these therapies to treat illness or maintain health. This book can increase healthcare professionals' ability to care for people as individuals and truly understand their comprehensive healthcare needs.

Carol P. Curtiss, RN, MSN
Clinical Specialist Consultant
Greenfield, MA
Past President, Oncology Nursing Society (1992–1993)

Eisenberg, D.M., Davis, R.B., Ettner, S.L., Appel, S., Wilkey, S., Van Rompay, M., & Kessler, R.C. (1998). Trends in alternative medicine use in the United States, 1990–1997: Results of a follow-up national survey. *JAMA, 280,* 1569–1575.

Porter-O'Grady, T. (1999, April 17). Keynote address, American Society of Pain Management Nurses Ninth Annual Meeting, Washington, DC.

A Short History of Medicine

2000 B.C. — "Here, eat this root."

1000 A.D. — "That root is heathen. Say this prayer."

1850 A.D. — "That prayer is superstition. Drink this potion."

1940 A.D. — "That potion is snake oil. Swallow this pill."

1985 A.D. — "That pill is ineffective. Take this antibiotic."

2000 A.D. — "That antibiotic doesn't work anymore. Here, eat this root."

—*Author unknown*

Introduction

Recent research documents the increased use of complementary and alternative therapies since 1990. At Integrative Care, the complementary therapy practice I founded, patients and healthcare professionals frequently ask, "But, where do I begin?" From these requests was born the concept for this book. It provides a place to begin. We have attempted to address the basic tenets of some of the most common therapies as well as descriptions of some lesser-known treatments while providing resources for ongoing reference.

My interest in complementary and alternative therapies began as a result of the inquiries of my patients. They taught me to think about these therapies with an open mind. They made me curious. I wanted to know more about the substances I saw on their kitchen counters when making home visits. I needed to know more about the therapies they described. The search for knowledge was fraught with limited and conflicting information.

The chapters in this book have been organized by categories of complementary and alternative therapies as defined by the National Institutes of Health (NIH), National Center for Complementary and Alternative Medicine. This format was chosen so that the information contained in the book would align with the published literature and information available on the Internet. All those concerned with this book have endeavored to make it easy to read and use. Typical of current culture, the information regarding these therapies is changing rapidly. Every effort, however, has been made to provide the most current information available at the time of publication.

Communication between healthcare professionals and patients must be enhanced. Misunderstandings occur when we speak to one another about therapies using terms that may have different meanings to different people. "Natural" does not mean "safe." Natural remedies and products can do harm unless taken or used in a prudent manner. There is much we do not know. It is, however, irresponsible, and perhaps unethical, for healthcare professionals to reject a therapy—and its potential benefits—simply because they are unfamiliar with it. Research has demonstrated that patients withhold information from their healthcare providers regarding their use of these therapies for a variety of reasons, including fear of dismissal. The communication between healthcare professionals and patients begins with mutual respect and is then augmented with open-mindedness and knowledge. Use of the term "alternative" when meaning "complementary" can be a source of misunderstanding and conflict. A therapy is alternative when it is used *instead of* conventional therapy. A therapy is complementary when it is used *in addition to* conventional therapy.

"Health" is being in a state of harmony. In today's world, we are under constant pressure and stress. It is increasingly difficult to attain or maintain balance and harmony. The impact of physical and emotional environments can be balanced by removing negative influence and strengthening the person. Central to this is the concept of holism; that is, physical, emotional, mental, and spiritual aspects of health are interconnected. The approach to attaining or restoring health cannot be a singular event or substance. Blending modalities offers healthcare professionals the opportunity to be holistic in the care of their patients.

Best wishes as you begin.

Georgia Decker

Georgia M. Decker, MS, RN, CS-ANP, AOCN
Editor

Chapter One

Mind-Body Interventions

Linda U. Krebs, RN, PhD, AOCN

Introduction

Mind-body medicine, which also is referred to as behavioral medicine, unites biomedical, behavioral, and psychosocial strategies for the promotion of health and the understanding of illness. Segen (1998) defined it as "an evolving field of health care based on the belief that a complex interplay of external and internal factors influence the mind, and therefore a person's response and recuperation from disease" (p. 243). Mind-body medicine is viewed as a holistic, healing philosophy predicated on the interconnection between the mind and body, the innate healing capacity of the body, and the potential for an individual to exercise some personal control over the healing process (Lewith, Kenyon, & Lewis, 1996). Basic principles of mind-body medicine include the beliefs that (a) each individual is unique; thus, the cause of disease and the strategies for cure and healing are unique and (b) chronic stress and lack of balance in one's life contribute to disease and illness (Burton Goldberg Group, 1993).

Although only recently gaining attention in Western medicine, mind-body interventions have been recognized for thousands of years by traditional medical systems. These interventions are based on the recognition that the mind and body are wholly integrated, each with the ability to influence the other. As described in the Workshop on Alternative Medicine (1994) report, "Mind-body relations are always mutual and bidirectional—the body affects the mind and is affected by it" (p. 4). A variety of interventions, including the use of relaxation techniques and creative art therapies, have been used to actively involve patients in their own treatment, thereby enhancing the body's inherent healing mechanisms and leading to altered expressions and experiences of illness for patients.

Controversy exists over whether mind-body interventions prolong survival or merely enhance quality of life and the sense of feeling healed (Cannistra, 1998). Anecdotal reports and individual case studies abound. Greer, Morris, and Pettingale (1979) noted that women with breast cancer who had a "fighting spirit" lived longer than those who felt helpless or hopeless. Recent literature has indicated that depression, stress, a lack of sense of control over life, a negative outlook, and a lack of social support correlate with poorer prognosis, while a sense of control, a positive outlook, and adequate social support are correlated with improved survival (Pelton & Overholser, 1994). What appears to be most important, however, is that patients place great value on feeling "healed" (defined as an enhanced sense of well-being, balance and harmony, and wholeness) even when cure is not attained and disease remains (Workshop on Alternative Medicine, 1994). For some, the use of mind-body interventions promotes this feeling.

Relaxation Techniques

Relaxation techniques include a variety of methods, such as biofeedback training, breath therapy, hypnotherapy, imagery and visualization, meditation, progressive muscle relaxation, and yoga, to reduce physical and mental stress. While the techniques vary in methodology, all require an environment that is free of distractions and that the participants attain a comfortable position and wear clothing that is nonrestrictive to movement and relaxation. The participant must be able to limit his or her focus to a single image, object, or phrase and must be able to attain a passive attitude of "letting go," thus allowing thoughts, fears, and concerns to be overcome (Segen, 1998).

Biofeedback Training

Biofeedback training is a component of autogenic training that was developed to allow an individual to gain voluntary control over processes within the body that previously were thought to be involuntary. Described in the early 1960s by Neal Miller, biofeedback training uses electronic equipment to assess and monitor a patient's ability to gain control over a symptom or function (Lewith, Kenyon, & Lewis, 1996). Once control is mastered, the patient is able to recognize early symptoms and take appropriate measures to minimize or alleviate them. A therapist (biofeedback trainer or practitioner) facilitates the process until the patient is able to achieve the desired results on his or her own.

In the initial phase of biofeedback training, an electronic device (i.e., an electrocardiogram, a temperature gauge, a blood pressure cuff, or a galvanic skin response indicator) is attached to an area of the body to "feed" responses to symptoms "back" to the patient. The measurement device continuously records and displays the response with a light or sound. With increased response, the light will brighten or the sound will become louder. Through a process of trial and error, and with the assistance of a biofeedback therapist, the patient will develop a method by which to individually alter the light or sound. With practice, the patient will be able to devise a method to totally extinguish the light or tone. Once this process is learned, the patient is then able to self-regulate behavior without the use of electronic equipment. Mastering the process typically takes 10–15 half-hour weekly sessions (Lewith et al., 1996). Recent technique updates have included the use of interactive software packages that allow the patient to learn to control images on a computer-based video display terminal (Woodham & Peters, 1997).

Biofeedback training has been used to decrease muscle tension and spasm, treat sleep disorders, control urinary and fecal incontinence, relieve chronic pain, and manage esophageal motility abnormalities. In patients with cancer, biofeedback training has been used alone or in conjunction with other therapies to prevent anticipatory nausea and vomiting, achieve pain relief, and decrease anxiety and stress related to disease and treatment (Kastner & Burroughs, 1993; Workshop on Alternative Medicine, 1994).

Special Considerations

No specific contraindications have been identified, and biofeedback appears to be safe for all patients. Patients are requested not to alter the doses of any medications without specific recommendations from their healthcare providers. Electrode sites should be monitored for local irritation (*Nurse's Handbook,* 1999). Success in using biofeedback is contingent upon patient motivation, the use of a competent therapist for biofeedback training, and a reasonable expectation that the use of biofeedback can alleviate the symptom or result in enhanced function (Segen, 1998).

Breath Therapy

Breath therapy, or breath regulation, consists of a number of techniques designed to increase energy that can be used to promote healing and self-care. Breathing techniques most commonly are combined with various methods of relaxation to enhance one's ability to cope with stress. Proper breathing is necessary for relaxation, to decrease tension, and to enhance calmness (Shealy, 1996). Strategies include the use of slow inhalation and exhalation to promote relaxation and forced respirations (also known as evocative breath therapy), which often is practiced with music and used to promote emotional release. Holotropic breathwork, or holotropic breathing, "combines breathing, evocative music, and a specific form of bodywork" (Kastner & Burroughs, 1993, p. 114). It combines the spiritual, physical, and psychological dimensions and is used to promote a sense of "wholeness."

When under stress, an individual may experience short, shallow breathing that can cause increased blood levels of carbon monoxide, leading to symptoms such as panic attacks, feeling faint, increased perspiration, muscle tension, and heart palpitations (Shealy, 1996; Woodham & Peters, 1997). Breath regulation therapies are intended to diminish or eliminate these symptoms. According to Shealy and Woodham and Peters, proper breathing techniques incorporate diaphragmatic, or abdominal, breathing.

Diaphragmatic breathing, which uses long, deep breaths that expand the rib cage, allows the respiratory system to function more efficiently because the lungs are entirely filled and emptied with each complete breath. This is particularly important because diaphragmatic breathing is associated with decreased stress, a sensation of calmness and well-being, and a state of relaxation and increased awareness of one's surroundings (Burton Goldberg Group, 1993; Woodham & Peters, 1997). A practitioner may be used to assist in mastery of proper breathing techniques.

Breath therapy has been used to decrease anxiety, pain, and stress (Ryder, 1997; Segen, 1998) and has been suggested to enhance immune function (Segen). Jahnke (1996) noted that proper breathing promotes homeostasis (balance) in the autonomic nervous system and may play a role in the movement of lymphatic fluid throughout the body.

Special Considerations

Breath therapy is contraindicated for patients who are experiencing shortness of breath.

Hypnotherapy

The beginnings of hypnotherapy can be traced to ancient Greeks and Egyptians, who used healing trances, and to aboriginal cultures in Africa and in North, Central, and South America, in which medicine men and women, shamans, and witch doctors created hypnotic states through drumming and dancing (Woodham & Peters, 1997). Franz Anton Mesmer, an 18th century Austrian physician, is believed to be the "founding father of hypnotherapy," although his peers considered him to be a charlatan (Kastner & Burroughs, 1993). Mesmer called his form of hypnotherapy "animal magnetism." James Baird, a Scottish surgeon, first used the term "hypnosis" in the 1840s; however, Milton H. Erickson is considered to be the "father of modern hypnotherapy" (Woodham & Peters). Sigmund Freud was an early proponent of hypnotherapy but later abandoned this method for his own forms of analysis (Burton Goldberg Group, 1993). Hypnotherapy has been considered a valid form of medical therapy since the early 1950s and is now widely used throughout the world (Shealy, 1996). A variety of forms have been postulated; the most common include (a) deep relaxation, in which stress is eased through relaxation, (b) suggestion therapy, which promotes positive thoughts and ideas, and (c) analytic therapy, which examines problems and their causes (Shealy).

Hypnotherapy has been described as a state of "heightened awareness" in which suggestions, as posed by the therapist or through autosuggestion (i.e., self-hypnosis), are more likely to be followed (Burton Goldberg Group, 1993). Through hypnotherapy, the body becomes relaxed and one's attention is focused on an image, an object, or other ideas as suggested by the therapist or oneself. The goal is to access the unconscious mind, which is believed to be less critical and more likely to accept suggestion. The use of imagery is central to hypnotherapy and may include mental images, sensory input, or words or thoughts. Shealy (1996) defined the hypnotic state as a "naturally occurring state of equilibrium somewhere between waking and sleeping" (p. 113).

For hypnotherapy to be beneficial, three conditions need to be present: (a) an affinity must exist between the patient and the hypnotherapist, (b) the environment must be suitable (comfortable and noise-free), and (c) the patient must be willing to be hypnotized. Individuals who attain the somnambulistic (deep) state of hypnotherapy are most likely to experience some benefit. The hypnotherapist serves as a facilitator, and self-hypnosis techniques can be taught for self-care (Burton Goldberg Group, 1993).

Approximately 90% of the population can be hypnotized; however, only 20%–30% can attain the somnambulistic state (Woodham & Peters, 1997). One cannot be hypnotized against one's will, and an individual will not follow suggestions unless he or she desires to do so (Woodham & Peters).

Hypnotherapy has been used successfully to alleviate stress; to decrease anxiety, depression, fear, and sensations of panic; and to treat headaches, migraines, addictions, bed-wetting, and sleep disorders (Arner, 1990; Segen, 1998). It has been noted to decrease blood pressure and respiratory rate and promote relaxation and a sense of well-being (Burton Goldberg Group, 1993). Hypnotherapy also has been used to manage addictions, enhance concentration, and manage stress-related illnesses (Shealy, 1996). In patients with cancer, hypnotherapy has been noted to diminish side effects related to cancer treatment and to control or decrease cancer pain (Segen; Spiegel & Moore, 1997). Gordon (1996) noted a decrease in nausea and vomiting, a 50% decrease in levels of pain, and an overall decrease in anxiety in patients with chemotherapy-related nausea and vomiting or cancer-related pain. Self-hypnosis has been used to ease pain and decrease chemotherapy-induced nausea and vomiting (Workshop on Alternative Medicine, 1994).

Special Considerations

Contraindications for the use of hypnotherapy include epilepsy, depression, organic psychiatric conditions, antisocial personality disorders, and severe psychosis (Burton Goldberg Group, 1993; Woodham & Peters, 1997). It is essential that a qualified therapist be used (see "Implications" section on page 23 for further details).

Imagery and Visualization

Techniques incorporating imagery and visualization (also referred to as guided imagery, creative imagery, or visualization therapy) use images or symbols to focus the mind on bodily functions. Gordon (1996) described imagery as a process that uses "the conscious mind to create mental images in order to evoke physiologic changes, promote natural healing processes, and provide insight and self-awareness" (p. 92). The goal is to create physiologic changes or to accomplish a particular goal (e.g., pain relief) through communicating positive thoughts about the desired outcome to the body (Kastner & Burroughs, 1993; Segen, 1998). Imagery is a common component of most mind-body therapies. The exact mechanism of action is unclear.

Florence Nightingale is suggested to have described imagery/visualization and its effects on health early in her career (Hoffart & Keene, 1998), while O. Carl Simonton pioneered imagery in the United States in the early 1970s (Gordon, 1996). Originally, this therapy incorporated aggressive images that consisted of waging war on, killing off, or eating up the symptom or problem. More recently, however, these aggressive images have been replaced by idyllic scenes and images of serenity and calm (Gordon, 1996).

Most techniques using imagery can be placed into one of three categories: (a) evaluation or diagnostic imagery, (b) mental rehearsal, and (c) therapeutic interventions. Therapeutic interventions are, by far, the most common (Workshop on Alternative Medicine, 1994). Phalen (1998) and Woodham and Peters (1997) described two forms of imagery: active and receptive. In active imagery, a particular image is selected by the patient and used to alter a situation or control a symptom. In receptive imagery, images that may provide information about the reasons for a particular symptom or problem are allowed to surface.

Imagery and visualization have been used to decrease stress, stage fright, tension, pain, headaches, and heart rate. Additionally, they have been noted to ameliorate symptoms related to premenstrual syndrome (PMS) and to assist patients in managing urinary incontinence (Burton Goldberg Group, 1993; Kastner & Burroughs, 1996). Guided imagery and visualization may stimulate the immune system (Segen, 1998). Patients with cancer have used imagery and visualization for relaxation and minimization or relief of treatment- and disease-related symptoms, for emotional release, to gain an understanding about the meaning of the cancer experience, and for pain relief (Rancour, 1994; Ryder, 1997). Troesch, Rodehaver, Delaney, and Yates (1993) randomized 40 patients who were receiving chemotherapy with cisplatin to two groups: conventional antiemetic therapy with or without the addition of guided imagery. Although they found no statistical differences in the occurrence of nausea, vomiting, and retching between the groups, patients using guided imagery reported feeling more in control and had a more positive view of the chemotherapy experience. In addition, the experimental group developed the most distressing symptoms at 48 hours, compared to within 12 hours for the control group. In another study, the combination of guided imagery and relaxation increased the ability to manage pain associated with oral mucositis in patients who were undergoing bone marrow transplant as compared to controls or those receiving support from a therapist (Syrjala, Donaldson, Davis, Kippes, & Carr, 1995).

Special Considerations

Few contraindications exist for the use of guided imagery except for patients who are known to be psychotic (*Nurse's Handbook,* 1999). However, in some instances, the image can trigger a physical response, such as an asthma attack when imaging a field of flowers. In addition, some patients may identify so completely with the image that the inability to accomplish the goal or solve the problem may be seen as failure (Cleaveland, 1997). Although imagery can be used as a self-help technique, because of the potential to evoke troubling or disturbing images, initial practice should begin under the guidance of a skilled therapist who has been educated in the art and science of imagery. It may be possible to enhance the effects of imagery by the addition of a smell, which may evoke the desired image for the patient (*Nurse's Handbook*).

Meditation

Meditation has been practiced for thousands of years and is a component of all cultures and every major religion (Kastner & Burroughs, 1993; Woodham & Peters, 1997). Meditation is viewed as a therapeutic method through which an individual is able to block out nonessential thoughts, raise the mind to a higher level, and, thus, transcend everyday concerns (Segen, 1998). Through meditation, one is believed to be able to come into contact with one's inner energy and emotions, calm the mind, relax the body, and concentrate on the moment (Gordon, 1996; Pelton & Overholser, 1994; Phalen, 1998). Meditation can involve breath awareness, repetitive movement, or the use of a mantra, a religious icon, or a physical object to achieve deep relaxation (Woodham & Peters).

Gordon (1996) described two basic approaches to meditation: concentrative meditation and mindfulness meditation. In concentrative meditation, one focuses attention on a sound, an image, or one's breathing, while in mindfulness meditation, the mind is allowed to remain open to whatever flows through. Kastner and Burroughs (1993) and Segen (1998) further categorized meditation techniques based on whether they involve the mind or the body or incorporate techniques for letting go or maintaining control. These include (a) control of the body through activities such as yoga, (b) control of the mind through visualizing an image, focusing on an object, or repeating a word or syllable, (c) letting go of the body through intentional release of muscle tension, and (d) letting go of the mind through leaving the mind open to new thoughts and ideas. As noted by Pelton and Overholser (1994), the meditation technique used is unique to the individual.

Transcendental meditation is the most widely known form of meditation in the United States. It is based on Hindu philosophy and was introduced to the United States in the 1950s by Maharishi Mahesh Yogi (Shealy, 1996). In transcendental meditation, a repeated mantra (sound or tone) is used to achieve deep relaxation and enhance mental clarity. Reported benefits include increased longevity and quality of life and decreased anxiety (Phelan, 1998; Shealy; Workshop on Alternative Medicine, 1994).

Meditation has been shown to be of benefit in decreasing blood pressure and lowering respiratory and heart rates (Gordon, 1996; Segen, 1998). It also has been noted to decrease insomnia, anger, aggression, and nervousness; relieve muscular aches and pains; and increase concentration and mental clarity (Phelan, 1998). In patients with cancer, meditation has been shown to have a calming effect with a resultant alleviation or decrease in pain, anxiety, and depression and decreased chemotherapy-related nausea (Murphy, Morris, & Lange, 1997; Ryder, 1997). Ainslie Meares, a psychiatrist in Melbourne, Australia, has suggested that meditation may increase blood flow, and thus oxygen and white blood cells, to the tumor (Pelton & Overholser, 1994).

Special Considerations

Individuals with epilepsy or schizophrenia should avoid practicing meditation because of reports of grand mal seizures in the former and acute psychotic events in the latter when meditation techniques were used (Gordon, 1996; *Nurse's Handbook*, 1999). In addition, the special considerations related to breathing, imagery, relaxation, and exercise should be reviewed if these methods are incorporated into the meditation process.

Relaxation Therapy/Progressive Muscle Relaxation

Shealy (1996) defined relaxation therapy as a method that "allows the mind-body complex to get on with its own healing work, restoring internal harmony, and creating afresh conditions for release of mental and physical tension" (p. 116). Breathing techniques are the foundation of relaxation, and most relaxation strategies begin by having participants focus on their patterns of breathing. Relaxation can be used in almost any setting, is easy to learn, and allows the patient to achieve maximal benefit in a minimal amount of time (Gordon, 1996; Woodham & Peters, 1997). Hiltebrand and Annala (1998) noted that relaxation is a simple, effective method for patients with cancer to manage symptoms associated with cancer and its treatments. As with many of the mind-body therapies, the benefits of relaxation have been known for thousands of years.

Most forms of relaxation include controlled breathing techniques combined with muscle relaxation, usually in the form of systematic tensing and relaxing of muscle groups. Pioneered by Edmund Jacobson in the 1930s, progressive muscle relaxation incorporates breathing to allow the participant to consciously relax skeletal muscles by initially tensing and then relaxing, or letting go of the tension, in the specific muscle group (Woodham & Peters, 1997). The process begins by tensing the feet and progressively moves up the body. Upon completion, all muscles, potentially even smooth, internal muscles, are relaxed; one feels as if the "idle" of the body's "engine" has been returned to normal (Bricklin, 1990; Gordon, 1996; Woodham & Peters).

Relaxation therapy has been used to decrease stress, anxiety, depression, blood pressure, and symptoms of PMS. In individuals with cancer, it may decrease pain, nausea, vomiting, and the stress and anxiety associated with diagnosis and treatment (Hiltebrand & Annala, 1998; Shealy, 1996; Woodham & Peters, 1997). Baider, Uziely, and De-Nour (1994) studied the impact of six sessions of progressive muscle relaxation and guided imagery on individuals with cancer. Of the 86 patients who completed the entire course, all experienced a decrease in symptoms and their impact on quality of life. Sloman, Brown, Aldana, and Chee (1994) and Sloman (1995) reported improved cancer pain relief in patients receiving relaxation training, with or without guided imagery. Additionally, Burish and Jenkins (1992) and Arakawa (1997) conducted studies that demonstrated significant decreases in nausea and anxiety in patients who received relaxation treatment. Finally, Wallace (1997) conducted a meta-analysis of published studies concerning relaxation and guided imagery interventions for cancer pain and found decreased distress and pain and increased physiologic functioning and visual concentration in patients who received these interventions.

Special Considerations

While assisting patients to relax does no harm and may be of benefit in reducing stress and alleviating feelings of helplessness (Kastner & Burroughs, 1993), contraindications do exist. Relaxation therapy is contraindicated in individuals who experience shortness of breath or who have experienced increased stress or anxiety when attempting to focus on breathing. Techniques that use progressive muscle relaxation with intermittent tensing and relaxing of muscles are contraindicated in individuals with bone metastases or compromised functional status. Therapy must be individualized to the unique needs and requirements of the patient (Hiltebrand & Annala, 1998; Shealy, 1996).

Yoga

Yoga is believed to have originated in India more than 5,000 years ago. Often called "the work," "the way," or "the path," yoga is based on ancient Indian Vedic teachings (Kastner & Burroughs, 1993) and traditionally was practiced by Hindu ascetics (yogis). Its name is derived from the Sanskrit *yuj*, which means "union," and the word *yoga* itself means to combine, coordinate, or harmonize. Yoga as it is known today is thought to be the product of Patanjali, who wrote the *Yoga Sutras* following a period of meditation in the mountains of India in 200 B.C. (Woodham &

Peters, 1997). It was introduced into the West in the 19th century and is considered to be a "fully integrated system controlling all aspects of life" (Woodham & Peters, p. 108). Gardner (1990) stated that the goal of yoga is to attain good health, which includes a simple diet, outdoor exercise, a tranquil mind, and an awareness of one's relationship with one's creator. She defined a healthy person as one who experiences unity of body, mind, and spirit. Because healing is believed to begin with relaxation, yoga also begins with a period of relaxation.

In its purest form, yoga consists of eight stages (limbs), each increasingly spiritual, to the attainment of enlightenment, or *samadhi*. The first four limbs consist of postures (*asanas*) and breathing exercises (*prana*, meaning "life energy") that are designed to purify and bring the body and mind into harmony. The second four consist of meditative practices that eventually lead to enlightenment. *Asanas* may be therapeutic or meditative and always are practiced with breath control exercises. They are designed to create bodily ease or comfort, to facilitate meditation, or as therapy for a specific physical symptom or disorder. *Samadhi* is attained only after dedicated and disciplined practice. When an individual has reached *samadhi*, he or she is believed to have gone beyond the normal states of consciousness (i.e., waking, dream, and sleep) to a fourth level (Lewith et al., 1996).

Many different types of yoga exist, ranging from yoga therapy used to maintain health or combat a specific medical problem to power yoga (*ashtanga*). In the Western world, the most common type is Hatha yoga, or health yoga. Hatha yoga is a technique for achieving better health through total care of the body and all of its functions. It is a combination of *asanas* and *pranayama* that, when practiced appropriately, leads to a calm mind, steady breathing, and a relaxed body. A minimum of one hour of practice per day is believed to be necessary to attain the suggested benefits. Regular daily practice enhances one's energy, stamina, muscle tone, and concentration, resulting in a greater sense of control and an improved ability to manage stress (Woodham & Peters, 1997).

Yoga has been shown to have a physiologic effect on circulation and muscle tone. Suggested uses include symptomatic relief of back pain, arthritis, stress, fatigue, asthma, bronchitis, PMS, anxiety, muscle tension, and a variety of other conditions, including cancer. The *asanas* are thought to affect the endocrine glands and autonomic nervous system, stimulating digestion, the lymphatic system, and brain activity (Gardner, 1990; Kastner & Burroughs, 1993; Segen, 1998; Shealy, 1996; Woodham & Peters, 1997). Anecdotal reports of 29 individuals with cancer suggested that 90% had some positive benefit from practicing yoga (Burton Goldberg Group, 1993).

Special Considerations

When practiced appropriately, yoga has no known side effects. One should exercise caution when attempting new postures. Certain postures, particularly headstands, should not be attempted during pregnancy or by patients with hypertension or heart disease. Individuals with diabetes, hernias, cancer metastatic to bone, or a history of eye, ear, or brain problems should consult with their healthcare providers prior to beginning any yoga program (Shealy, 1996; Woodham & Peters, 1997).

Qigong

Qigong is an ancient Chinese form of exercise that, similar to yoga, incorporates breathing exercises, movement, and meditation. In conjunction with other components of Chinese traditional medicine, Qigong has been used to reduce stress and maintain health through balancing the body's energy along identified meridians that correspond to the body's emotions and organs (Phalen, 1998). The goal of Qigong is to influence the flow of qi, the vital life energy or animating force of the body. Abnormalities of qi are evidenced as stagnation, collapse, deficiency, and rebellion (Beinfield & Korngold, 1995). The two primary branches (forms) of Qigong include soft (internal) Qigong, in which the qi is self-manipulated through various forms of exercise and breathing techniques, and hard (external) Qigong, in which the qi is extended to another (i.e., one uses his or her energy to heal another) (Beinfield & Korngold; Segen, 1998). Additional branches include static Qigong, which involves minimal or no movement, and dynamic Qigong, which incorporates movement. Although multiple branches of Qigong exist, all include specific activities designed to regulate the body, the mind, and breathing. Additional forms may incorporate some form of automassage or extremity and torso movement that includes both gentle stretching and circular movements. These exercises may be done while sitting, standing, or lying down; body positioning is dependent upon the expected outcome of the individual exercise (Gordon, 1996; Kastner & Burroughs, 1993).

Qigong has been stated to be of benefit in managing gastrointestinal complaints, reducing stress and fatigue, improving circulation, improving resistance to disease, and decreasing blood pressure, pulse, respiratory rate, and oxygen consumption through providing emotional release and a sense of serenity. Some also have suggested that the practice of Qigong can bolster immune function and may prolong survival in individuals with cancer and HIV/AIDS (Burton Goldberg Group, 1993; Segen, 1998; Woodham & Peters, 1997).

Special Considerations

No known side effects or contraindications have been identified; however, individuals with bone tumors or metastases or those with severe bone marrow depression should contact their healthcare providers prior to attempting any aspect of Qigong.

Creative Arts Therapies

The creative arts therapies, consisting of art, dance, drama, music, sound, and other related forms of expression, have played an integral part in healing and self-expression. In many instances, emotions and reactions to illness may be expressed nonverbally earlier and with less difficulty than possible with verbal forms of expression. Creative arts therapies can foster healing, offer clarity to feelings and emotions, increase insight, and make concrete the vague, unexplainable feelings often related to illness and treatment (Hedlund, 1998; Kastner & Burroughs, 1993; Woodham & Peters, 1997).

Art Therapy

Art therapy is the use of drawing, painting, sculpture, or other creative forms for therapeutic benefit. It is designed to improve, maintain, or restore mental or physical well-being through nonverbal expression and communication. It provides a means through which patients can express unspoken concerns about their illnesses and reconcile emotional conflict. Art therapy's origins can be traced to the 1800s with the work of Rudolf Steiner, who proposed art as a method of healing (Woodham & Peters, 1997), but it was not defined as a profession until 1915, when Margaret Naumberg founded the Walden School, where she incorporated the use of art to meet her students' psychological needs (Kastner & Burroughs, 1993). Art therapy has been used with war veterans as a form of post-traumatic rehabilitation, is being investigated as a tool in patients with Alzheimer's disease to promote free expression, is widely used for personal development, and is used by patients with cancer to assist in adapting and coping with disease- and treatment-related sequelae (Segen, 1998; Woodham & Peters, 1997; Workshop on Alternative Medicine, 1994).

Art therapy can incorporate any art form, from painting to pottery to arts and crafts and model making. In many instances, the actual act of creating a product is therapeutic, whereas in other instances, the product tells a story or has symbolic meaning that may be analyzed and discussed to facilitate healing. Art may be used as a vehicle for expressing socially unacceptable emotions, such as jealousy or rage, or socially acceptable but sometimes personally unacceptable feelings, such as fear, grief, and confusion. As a method of self-help, art therapy can allow an individual to convey thoughts and feelings, relax, and release emotions. By drawing themselves, some patients with cancer find that they can more readily express their feelings about disease, treatment, and survival (Workshop on Alternative Medicine, 1994).

Art therapy is believed to be of benefit for managing stress, bereavement, mental and emotional illness, anorexia nervosa, low self-esteem, Alzheimer's disease, and terminal illness. Many patients with cancer have used art therapy to describe their reactions to and feelings about diagnosis, treatment, and stages of survival and as a method of healing (Hedlund, 1998; Hiltebrand & Annala, 1998; Kastner & Burroughs, 1993; Segen, 1998; Woodham & Peters, 1997). Patients with cancer who are experiencing pain have found that drawing portraits that depict themselves with and without pain has been helpful in understanding cancer pain and easing the pain experience (Pimentel, 1998).

Special Considerations

Art therapy has the potential to elicit unexpected responses triggered by the release of emotions; thus, it is recommended that a qualified and registered therapist be available to help the patient to deal with these emotions. No contraindications to the use of art therapy in individuals with cancer have been described, although a patient's physical status and medications must be taken into consideration when planning projects.

Dance Therapy

Dance therapy, or dance movement therapy, assists individuals to become aware of and express feelings and emotions with a goal of building self-esteem, regaining a sense of identity, and restoring or improving balance between mind and body. Marian Chase developed dance therapy in the United States in the 1940s as a method of expressing one's self through movement. In 1966, the American Dance Therapy Association was founded (Workshop on Alternative Medicine, 1994).

Dance therapy functions on the premise that, through the use of rhythm and movement, the conscious mind can be bypassed and contact can be made with the inner emotional world. Through dance, patients can learn to adapt to disabilities, cope with change, and express emotions and feelings. Dance therapy may be performed with or without a therapist. When a therapist is used, movement may either be choreographed or spontaneous, and music is not required. A typical "session" includes a warm-up and then finger and hand movements that eventually progress to involvement of the entire body. Props often are used but are not required. Simple steps, including walking, sliding, and swaying, are incorporated into the dance. Additionally, classical ballet movements may be incorporated to promote body flexibility, symmetrical movement, good posture, and balance (Kastner & Burroughs, 1993; Segen, 1998; Woodham & Peters, 1997).

Aerobic dance, created by Jackie Sorenson in 1970, and Jazzercise, created by Judie Sheppard Missett in 1969, are two of the many more specialized forms of dance therapy. Each of these forms is considered to be a complete physical-fitness and body-conditioning program that incorporates dance movements with basic exercises. Tribal dancing, used for thousands of years by aborigines and other indigenous peoples, also can be used as dance therapy. It promotes mental and physical relaxation, provides exercise, and develops participant unity into a tightly woven social community (Kastner & Burroughs, 1993; Workshop on Alternative Medicine, 1994).

Dance therapy is believed to be of benefit for individuals with anorexia nervosa, bulimia, learning disabilities, stress, tension, anxiety, and depression. For women with breast cancer, dance therapy may be used to increase range of motion on the affected side, increase flexibility, decrease lymphedema, and increase self-esteem and self-confidence (Davis, 1998).

Special Considerations

Although no contraindications have been described for the use of dance therapy, individuals at risk for pathologic fractures or those experiencing peripheral neuropathies in the feet and lower extremities should be cautioned about falls and the potential for injury. The potential for cardiovascular compromise from strenuous activity should be evaluated prior to beginning dance therapy. A qualified, registered therapist is recommended. Dance therapy does have the potential to elicit unexpected responses triggered by the release of emotions (Burton Goldberg Group, 1993; Woodham and Peters, 1997).

Drama Therapy

Drama therapy is the deliberate use of the theater arts for therapeutic benefit. Ranging from theater productions to puppetry and mime, drama therapy is designed to release emotions, allow for free expression, promote symptom relief, and support personal growth through active participation. An important aspect of drama therapy is the use of improvisational techniques that allow for free expression and exploration of feelings and the playing-out of experiences and unsettling events. Drama therapy also can promote change though exploration and dramatization (i.e., role-play) of potential events and conflicts (Kastner & Burroughs, 1993).

Drama therapy may be of benefit in those who are experiencing emotional trauma, stressful life events, and depression and for those who are developmentally disabled, are elderly, or have cancer or HIV/AIDS.

Special Considerations

The potential exists for eliciting unexpected responses triggered by the release of emotions; thus, the availability of a qualified and registered therapist is recommended. No known contraindications have been described.

Music Therapy

For more than 2,000 years, music has been known to have therapeutic benefits (Bricklin, 1990; Woodham & Peters, 1997). Aristotle (ca. fourth century BC) believed that flute playing provided healing, and Pythagoras (ca. sixth century BC) believed that music, along with diet, was a primary means to promote health and harmony in mind and body (Bricklin; Kastner & Burroughs, 1993; Workshop on Alternative Medicine, 1994). In 400 BC, European Christians used chanting and intonation to treat illness. Music has been shown to decrease tension, facilitate the release of emotions, and provide an avenue for the exploration of thoughts and concerns (Shealy, 1996, Woodham & Peters).

Music therapy is the intentional use of music or sound (i.e., using an instrument [including the voice], writing music, or listening to music) to induce health and healing. It has been noted to be an effective nonverbal method of exploring and expressing feelings that have not previously or easily been put into words (Segen, 1998; Shealy, 1996; Woodham & Peters, 1997). Music may be stimulative, encouraging movement and participation (e.g., Gospel, Big Band, Dixieland), or sedative, promoting serenity and relaxation (e.g., classical compositions) (Segen).

The National Association for Music Therapy, Inc. was founded in 1950. Music therapists observe and assess patients, develop and initiate a plan of therapy, and evaluate therapeutic outcomes. They may work with individual patients or conduct music therapy group sessions. Group work often promotes the development of trust that may facilitate emotional expression. Therapy is individualized to the person or group and is based on personal or group preferences and surrounding environment (Workshop on Alternative Medicine, 1994). Cleaveland (1997) suggested that music therapy sessions allow a minimum of 20 minutes for listening or participating in a music-related activity in order to achieve optimum effects.

Sound therapy is a subset of music therapy that involves the use of sound waves to restore body harmony. It may incorporate chanting or toning, in which elongated vowel sounds are made and allowed to resonate throughout the body. These practices are believed to decrease stress and create harmony between mind and body, although no specific research findings to support this could be found. Recently, the use of a musical bed, with speakers that amplify musical vibrations transmitted through a mattress, has been suggested.

Music therapy has been used with individuals who are experiencing anxiety, depression, insomnia, low self-esteem, and communication disorders. In patients with Alzheimer's disease, specific types of music have evoked memories and facilitated recall (Burton Goldberg Group, 1993). In patients with cancer, music therapy has been shown to decrease the need for analgesics (Beck, 1991), promote emotional release, increase communication, decrease tension and feelings of helplessness, and increase verbal interactions (Lane, 1992; Ryder, 1997). Ezzone, Baker,

Rosselet, and Terepka (1998) randomized 39 patients who were undergoing high-dose chemotherapy for bone marrow transplant to receive either conventional antiemetic therapy or conventional therapy plus a music therapy intervention. The researchers noted that patients in the experimental group experienced a statistically significant decrease in nausea and vomiting as compared with patients in the control group. Emma O'Brien, BMUS, RMT, a music therapist from the Royal Melbourne Hospital in Melbourne, Australia, has used music therapy to assist patients in defining the cancer experience and in coping with disease and treatment. A CD, *Life Sounding the Soul*, using materials written by or for individual patients was produced and has been used in both therapeutic and educational settings. Patient ratings of their music therapy experiences have shown benefit (i.e., increased comfort and decreased side effects) in both the acute-care and palliative-care settings (E. O'Brien, personal communication, December 3,1998).

Special Considerations

No contraindications to music therapy have been described. The potential to elicit unexpected responses triggered by releasing emotions exists; thus, the availability of a qualified and registered therapist is recommended. O'Brien (personal communication, December 3, 1998) reported that release of emotions is not uncommon and is felt to be therapeutic by most patients and care providers.

Poetry Therapy

Poetry therapy (also known as bibliotherapy), developed by Eli Grifer in the 1940s, is the planned use of poetry or other forms of literature to elicit or clarify emotions, release stress, resolve conflict, and promote personal growth. Poetry therapy may include individual, creative forms of expression or the discussion and analysis of another's work. Although often conducted in a group with a poetry therapist, reading or writing of poetry and other forms of literature on one's own may provide an avenue for the expression of emotions that one may find difficult to express verbally. Poetry used in group sessions is chosen for a specific effect or to elicit certain types of responses; metaphors and analogies may be used. The reading, writing, and analysis of all forms of literature was noted to be of benefit to prisoners of Nazi concentration camps, who used poetry and storytelling to preserve their sanity and sense of humanity (Kastner & Burroughs, 1993).

Poetry therapy may be of benefit for individuals with anorexia nervosa, bulimia, Alzheimer's disease, stress, depression, strokes, or emotional trauma. In the elderly, poetry therapy may evoke memories and foster communication with others. In patients with cancer, expression through poetry and other forms of writing has been shown to decrease stress, reduce trauma related to disease and treatment, clarify emotional responses, and promote healing. In some instances, the sharing of writings with others has opened the doors of communication between families and friends, increasing quality of life (Heiney, 1995).

Special Considerations

No contraindications to poetry therapy have been described. However, side effects include the potential to elicit unexpected responses triggered by releasing emotions; thus, the availability of a qualified and registered therapist is recommended.

Other Therapies

Many other well-known mind-body therapies exist. Among these are myriad psychotherapy techniques and support groups. Additionally, horticultural therapy, pet therapy, and the use of prayer and spirituality, although in existence for many years, are gaining increased interest.

Horticultural Therapy

Horticultural therapy, as defined by Morgan (1989), "uses gardening, plants, floral materials, and vegetation to stimulate clients' interest in their surroundings and to promote the development of leisure or vocational skills" (p. 15). Plants have been used therapeutically since colonial times, with the first description presented by Benjamin Rush in the 1770s (Smith, 1998). The first known greenhouse created for horticultural therapy was built in Pennsylvania in 1879 (Smith). Horticultural therapy includes projects ranging from designing, planting, and tending a garden, flower bed, or potted plant to making potpourri, painting pumpkins, or making grapevine wreaths (Morgan). As an adjunct therapy, horticultural therapy primarily has been used with individuals with chronic mental-health problems or with those who are socially isolated. Horticultural therapy has been used in children's rehabilitation centers, with the elderly, and in intergenerational programs. Benefits include decreased aggression and anxiety, increased socialization, and an enhanced sense of well-being (Smith).

Although not described for use with individuals with cancer, the potential to be creative, to promote a futures orientation, and to relieve stress and anxiety suggests that horticultural therapy could be beneficial for this patient population.

Special Considerations

Contraindications to this therapy exist for those who are severely immunocompromised. Those who are at risk for or currently afflicted with lymphedema should use appropriate arm and hand care.

Pet Therapy

Pet therapy is the use of domesticated animals for therapeutic purposes. Dogs are the most commonly involved pets, although cats, horses, birds, fish, and other animals also have been used. For inpatient visits, animals are washed and groomed prior to visiting the patients. Some animals are specifically trained so that they can be taken to visit patients in nursing homes and mental institutions as well as to schools to visit children with specialized educational needs. These animals often act as ice breakers, assisting therapists to communicate with clients (Bricklin, 1990).

Pets provide love, warmth, and security, and individuals often respond better to them than other human beings (Bricklin, 1990). Exposure to pets helps many individuals to express emotions that they previously were unable to express and may open lines of communication. Having pets also has been shown to be therapeutic, providing both physical benefits (through such activities as walking a dog) and emotional benefits (through unconditional love and a sense of being needed) (Ryder, 1997).

Pet therapy has been shown to decrease social isolation, decrease stress and anxiety, provide a sense of comfort and support, and decrease heart and respiratory rates and blood pressure. For example, patients with cancer are thought to experience a calming sensation when exposed to aquariums, and the act of taking care of pets has been associated with decreasing one's sense of loneliness and isolation and providing a sense of control over part of one's life (Ryder, 1997).

Special Considerations

Side effects include the possibility of allergic reactions, bites, and scratches. No specific contraindications have been described except for those with known allergies. Those with severe bone marrow suppression probably should limit their exposure to animals. Animals should be examined thoroughly by a veterinarian and bathed and brushed prior to any patient visit.

Prayer

Prayer as a technique for healing has multiple components and varies widely from culture to culture. Prayer may be integral to a patient's life prior to an illness and, thus, continued through diagnosis, treatment, and follow-up, or it may become a component of an individual's self-help plan following diagnosis or the development of initial symptoms. Prayer for the sick includes asking a higher power to cure, promote healing, or relieve suffering of another individual. Many ill individuals, including patients with cancer, have visited healing shrines, such as Lourdes in the south of France, the Basilica of Our Lady of Guadeloupe in Mexico, and Compostele in Spain, in the hopes of finding a miraculous cure or some form of healing (Segen, 1998). Montbriand (1993, 1994) noted that patients often recite sets of prayers, usually asking St. Jude, the patron saint of hopeless causes, to intercede on their behalf.

For many, prayer has a calming effect and is used to provide a sense of support and safety (Ryder, 1997). In a study by Nokes, Kendrew, and Longo (1995), prayer was noted to be the fourth most common complementary therapy used by individuals with HIV/AIDS. In the majority of cases, it was used daily. Prayer can alleviate stress, assist in adapting and coping with illness, decrease vital signs, and allow for release of emotions. It also has been said to decrease symptoms (including decreases in pain, nausea, vomiting, and anxiety), provide a sense of being healed, and even induce spontaneous remission or cure from cancer (Dossey, 1996; Krebs, 1997; Larsen & Milano, 1995; Marwick, 1995; Segen, 1998).

Spirituality and prayer play important roles in healing. Completing a patient-focused spiritual assessment allows the healthcare provider to assess an individual patient's identified meaning and purpose in life, inner strengths, and ability to connect with others in life-giving ways (Dossey, 1998). The report from the Workshop on Alternative Medicine (1994) identified numerous studies that used prayer, or "prayerfulness," either locally or from a distance, to promote healing. The participants could derive no firm conclusions from the findings; they recommended further investigations into this arena. Dossey and Dossey (1998) noted that more than 250 published studies show that religious practices, regardless of type, are beneficial for health and healing. In addition, Brown-Saltzman (1997) noted that prayers can be worthwhile approaches that nurses can use when caring for patients with cancer.

Special Considerations

No specific side effects or contraindications have been ascribed to prayer therapy, although an individual may feel guilty if he or she prays, leads a spiritual life, or is prayed for and healing or cure does not occur.

Psychotherapy

Psychotherapy is a "catch-all" term used to describe therapy for behavioral, psychiatric, emotional, and personality disorders through verbal and nonverbal methods of communication. The most well-known form of psychotherapy is classical psychotherapy, which is based on the Freudian school of psychoanalysis. In general, psychotherapy is less intense than psychoanalysis and is more interactive, with the therapist providing advice and encouragement (Segen, 1998).

Multiple forms of psychotherapy exist, including therapies that rely on verbal communication, those that focus on changing perceptions and habits, and those that encourage patients to explore and take responsibility for their own actions. These include four major types: (a) the psychoanalytic therapies, which emanate from Freudian principles and attempt to understand current behaviors and ideas by understanding memories that lie in the unconscious mind, (b) counseling techniques, which focus on the management of a specific problem or life crisis, (c) behavioral therapies, which focus on altering negative behaviors and emotions, and (d) humanistic therapies, which assist participants to understand and take responsibility for their own thoughts and emotions (Shealy, 1996; Woodham & Peters, 1997; Workshop on Alternative Medicine, 1994). Within each major type, numerous specific therapies exist, each with its own defined set of principles and methods to promote emotional and physical well-being. Therapies may be undertaken individually or as part of a group.

Therapists involved in psychotherapy include psychoanalysts, psychologists, psychotherapists, counselors, social workers, nurses, and a variety of other specially accredited and credentialed individuals. Education and training can range from years of advanced education and clinical practice, including personal exposure to psychotherapeutic techniques, to a weekend or two of training. The role of the therapist includes evaluation of the problem, followed by the provision of individualized advice and encouragement that leads to resolution of the problem or adjustment to the situation. The therapist primarily functions as a sounding board, facilitating discussion that allows clients to solve their own problems (Segen, 1998; Woodham & Peters, 1997).

In addition to decreasing anxiety, increasing a sense of control, and enhancing the ability to cope with disease and treatment (Fawzy, Fawzy, Arndt, & Pasnau, 1995; Horrigan, 1995; Woodham & Peters, 1997; Workshop on Alternative Medicine, 1994), psychotherapeutic interventions also may increase the life expectancy of patients with cancer. Simonton, Matthews-Simonton, and Sparks (1980) noted that patients using psychotherapy in addition to conventional cancer treatment had double the survival time of those who did not participate in psychotherapy. Lawrence LeShan, as described in an interview with Horrigan, began psychotherapeutic interventions with patients with cancer in 1952. At that time, the medical paradigm for psychotherapy focused on what was wrong with the patient. LeShan noted that this type of therapy did not seem to be particularly beneficial to his patients. He subsequently changed his focus to evaluate what the patient was doing right and how the patient could move on with life despite the reality of the situation. In evaluating his patients following this change in approach, LeShan noted that while prior long-term survival was less than 5%, almost 50% were experiencing long-term remissions with his new method and that many patients seemed to respond better to all forms of therapy (Horrigan).

Special Considerations

No contraindications to psychotherapy have been identified for individuals with cancer. Of highest importance is receiving therapy from an appropriately educated therapist who is capable of providing the type of therapy that is most needed by the individual patient.

Support Groups

Support groups, or mutual aid groups, are designed to provide social support to individuals with a common concern. Their primary goals are to aid individuals in finding meaning, creating a sense of belonging through group participation, and decreasing physical and emotional discomfort (Cella & Yellen, 1993; Pelton & Overholser, 1994). As an integral component of our social fabric, support groups promote coping with illness through facilitating communication, emotional release, peer support, decreased feelings of social isolation, and the development of a sense of value for one's life experiences (Murphy et al., 1997; Pilisuk, Wentzel, Barry, & Tennant, 1997). Support groups have been shown to enhance physical and emotional adjustment to disease with a concomitant decrease in treatment- and disease-related side effects (Meyer & Mark, 1995). Groups offer peer support, advice and counsel, and emotional support in an atmosphere in which participants can draw strength from one other. Through group interaction, participants may become empowered to gain or maintain a positive attitude and may learn new coping skills. Additionally, the opportunity exists for gaining new friendships, developing a sense of community, sharing fears and concerns in a supportive environment, mourning the loss of a loved one or one's own pending death, managing family relationships, and celebrating survival (Pelton & Overholser; Phalen, 1998; Pilisuk et al.).

Three support programs of note are The Wellness Community, Bernie Siegel's Exceptional Cancer Patients (EcaP), and the assorted support programs of the American Cancer Society. The Wellness Community was founded by Harold Benjamin in 1982 and is designed to foster health and well-being through patients helping patients. It is designed to be complementary to Western medical practices and includes individual and group support structures, education on self-help techniques and diet and nutrition, and social events. EcaP "is based on the principles of *carefrontation,* a loving, safe, therapeutic confrontation that facilitates personal change and healing" (Phalen, 1998, p. 72). The aim of EcaP is to assist patients to become "exceptional" patients with cancer—those who become well against all predicted odds. EcaP founder Siegel has noted that some patients become unexpectedly well (Phalen). Controversy exists concerning the potential to "blame the victim" (i.e., place the guilt or blame for not being cured on the individual with cancer) as opposed to assisting the individual to assume responsibility for his or her ability to heal (Phalen). The American Cancer Society's support programs are well-documented and include, but are not limited to, Reach to Recovery, I Can Cope™, and Look Good . . . Feel Better™ (Murphy et al., 1997).

In patients with cancer, the benefits of support groups have been shown not only through enhanced coping and vigor and decreased anxiety, tension, and confusion but also through enhanced survival and decreased death rates (Cella & Yellen, 1993; Murphy et al., 1997; Ryder, 1997). Spiegel and Moore (1997) reported a doubling in length of survival (36.6 months vs. 18.8 months) in women with metastatic breast cancer who participated in a year-long support group as compared to the control group. These women believed that they had gained so much from the group that they chose to continue to meet beyond the one-year experimental period. Additionally, in a study by Fawzy et al. (1993), patients with melanoma who participated in support groups had decreased recurrence rates (7 of 34 vs. 13 of 34) and decreased death rates (3 of 34 vs. 10 of 34) over the six-year study period.

Support groups have been noted to decrease anxiety, tension, feelings of confusion and helplessness/hopelessness, and fatigue and to impart a sense of vigor on participants (Richardson et al., 1997). They facilitate coping and communication and have been shown to enhance survival in patients with malignant melanoma and metastatic breast cancer.

The potential exists to create a release of emotions that cannot be adequately supported without the benefit of a qualified group leader. Although no contraindications for participation in support groups have been identified, those with emotional instability, schizophrenia, or any severe mental imbalance probably should not participate.

Implications

While there are few contraindications to the various therapies described under the category of mind-body medicine, numerous implications exist for nursing practice. Of extreme importance is ensuring that the patient receives the therapeutic intervention or education for self-help from a qualified therapist. While no rigid set of criteria exists to identify a "qualified" therapist (practitioner), there are some specific questions that can be asked and guidelines to follow to facilitate selection of a qualified therapist. These include:

1. Adequate education/training: All of the therapeutic interventions described in this section have national or international organizations that prescribe specific educational and/or training requirements. The therapist should meet these requirements. Additionally, the therapist should have received this education/training from a reputable institution.

2. Certification: If a specific certification is available for the intervention, the therapist preferably should hold that certification.
3. Membership in a professional organization: Because specific criteria are established for the professional organizations, membership may be an additional indicator of the therapist's qualifications.
4. Special qualifications: For specific therapies such as hypnosis or psychotherapy, the therapist should be licensed or otherwise appropriately educated and credentialed (e.g., MD, DDS, APN, LCSW).
5. Additional questions: The therapist also should describe the location and length of his or her training, length of practice, previous experience(s) with specific types of illness, previous success rates and problem/complication rates, and certification and compliance with the appropriate regulatory agency associated with that specific therapeutic intervention (Shealy, 1996; Woodham & Peters, 1997).

Many of these interventions will be undertaken by the patient as a form of self-help or may be suggested by a healthcare provider to assist in coping with disease or treatment. Numerous patients (and family members) keep journals, draw, paint, or use other forms of creative expression to describe their emotions related to diagnosis, treatment, and their sequelae. Additionally, patients may follow directions outlined in self-help books or audio- or videotapes or provided by members of the healthcare team to learn such practices as relaxation and guided imagery. This makes it imperative that the nurse be aware of any contraindications or potential complications and intervene appropriately. In addition to not forcing a patient to participate in an activity and recognizing that many of the mind-body medicine interventions have the potential to elicit strong emotions that may require specific and rapid medical interventions, the nurse should

1. Ensure that the patient is physically fit to undertake the desired activity through a thorough evaluation of the patient's medical/psychoemotional history and relevant physical examination. If any questions arise, the patient should be referred to the appropriate healthcare professional prior to undertaking the activity.
2. Educate the patient to continue with regularly prescribed medications and treatments.
3. Properly educate about and assess the patient for potential complications associated with a specific mind-body intervention and be prepared to intervene as needed.
4. Be able to identify additional resources that may be of benefit (e.g., support groups, qualified therapists).
5. Be aware of potential ethical issues (e.g., unqualified therapists, use of prayer or mental healing by others without the patient's knowledge).

6. Be aware of others in surrounding areas who may be affected (positively and negatively) by the therapeutic intervention and minimize intrusion.

7. Continue to provide routine care and other interventions as would be expected for that particular patient.

Summary

Mind-body interventions have been used for thousands of years by traditional medical systems and have become more widely used in Western medicine over the last several decades. Encompassing relaxation techniques, creative therapies, various forms of psychotherapy, and therapies using plants and animals, mind-body therapies generally are without contraindications for the typical patient. When practiced appropriately, with a qualified therapist or as self-care following adequate instruction, these therapies can help to alleviate symptoms and promote an increased sense of control, self-esteem, and quality of life.

References

Arakawa, S. (1997). Relaxation to reduce nausea, vomiting and anxiety induced by chemotherapy in Japanese patients. *Cancer Nursing, 20,* 342–349.

Arner, B.J. (1990). Hypnosis. In M. Bricklin (Ed.), *The practical encyclopedia of natural healing* (pp. 295–298). New York: Penguin Books.

Baider, L., Uziely, B., & De-Nour, A.K. (1994). Progressive muscle relaxation and guided imagery in cancer patients. *General Hospital Psychiatry, 16,* 340–347.

Beck, S.L. (1991). The therapeutic use of music for cancer-related pain. *Oncology Nursing Forum, 18,* 1327–1337.

Beinfield, H., & Korngold, E. (1995). Chinese traditional medicine: An introductory overview. *Alternative Therapies, 1*(1), 44–52.

Bricklin, M. (Ed.). (1990). *The practical encyclopedia of natural healing.* New York: Penguin Books.

Brown-Saltzman, K. (1997). Replenishing the spirit by meditative prayer and guided imagery. *Seminars in Oncology Nursing, 13,* 255–259.

Burish, T.G., & Jenkins, R.A. (1992). Effectiveness of biofeedback and relaxation training in reducing the side effects of cancer chemotherapy. *Health Psychology, 11*(1), 17–23.

Burton Goldberg Group. (1993). *Alternative medicine: The definitive guide.* Puyalluo, WA: Future Medicine Publishing.

Cannistra, S.A. (Ed.). (1998). Can the mind fight cancer? *Cancer Smart, 4*(1), 9.

Cella, D.F., & Yellen, S.B. (1993). Cancer support groups: The state of the art. *Cancer Practice, 1*(1), 56–61.

Cleaveland, M.J. (1997). Alternative therapies. In R.A. Gates & R.M. Fink (Eds.), *Oncology nursing secrets* (pp. 85–90). St. Louis: Mosby.

Davis, S.L. (1998). Dance therapy for the breast cancer survivor and how you can do it on your own. *Coping, 12*(1), 30.

Dossey, B. (1998). Holistic modalities & healing moments. *American Journal of Nursing, 98*(6), 44–47.

Dossey, B., & Dossey, L. (1998). Attending to holistic care. *American Journal of Nursing, 98*(8), 35–38.

Dossey, L. (1996). *Prayer as a healing force* [Online]. Available: www.healthy.net/hwlibraryarticles/mindbodyconnectio/dosseyw.htm [1997, December 31].

Ezzone, S., Baker, C., Rosselet, R., & Terepka, E. (1998). Music as an adjunct to antiemetic therapy. *Oncology Nursing Forum, 25,* 1551–1556.

Fawzy, F.I., Fawzy, N.W., Arndt, L.A., & Pasnau, R.O. (1995). Critical review of psychosocial interventions in cancer care. *Archives of General Psychiatry, 52*(2), 100–113.

Fawzy, F.I., Fawzy, N.W., Hyun, C.S., Elashoff, R., Guthrie, D., Fahey, J.L., & Morton, D.L. (1993). Malignant melanoma: Effects of an early structured psychiatric intervention, coping, and affective state on recurrence and survival 6 years later. *Archives of General Psychiatry, 50,* 681–689.

Gardner, T. (1990). Yoga therapy. In M. Bricklin (Ed.), *The practical encyclopedia of natural healing* (pp. 521–530). New York: Penguin Books.

Gordon, J.S. (1996). *Manifesto for a new medicine: Your guide to healing partnerships and the wise use of alternative therapies.* Reading, MA: Addison-Wesley.

Greer, S., Morris, T., & Pettingale, K.W. (1979). Psychological response to breast cancer: Effect on outcome. *Lancet, 2*(8146), 785–787.

Halsell, G. (1983). Visualization. In M. Bricklin (Ed.), *The practical encyclopedia of natural healing* (pp. 510–516). New York: Penguin Books.

Hedlund, S. (1998). More than a thousand words: Confronting cancer through art. *Coping, 12*(1), 48–49.

Heiney, S.P. (1995). The healing power of story. *Oncology Nursing Forum, 22,* 899–904.

Hiltebrand, E.U., & Annala, S. (1998, January/February). Adjunctive psychosocial support services as a complement to traditional interventions for the cancer population. *Cancer Management,* pp. 20–28.

Hoffart, M.B., & Keene, E.P. (1998). The benefits of visualization. *American Journal of Nursing, 98*(12), 44–47.

Horrigan, B. (1995). Larry LeShan: Mobilizing the life force, treating the individual. *Alternative Therapies in Health and Medicine, 1*(1), 63–69.

Jahnke, R. (1996). *Relaxation practices* [Online]. Available: www.healthy.net/library/books/jahnke/breath.htm [1997, December 31].

Kastner, M., & Burroughs, H. (1993). *Alternative healing.* LaMesa, CA: Halcyon Publishing.

Krebs, L.U. (1997). *Recreating harmony: Stories of Native American women surviving breast cancer.* Ann Arbor, MI: UMI Dissertation Services.

Lane, D. (1992). Music therapy: A gift beyond measure. *Oncology Nursing Forum, 19,* 863–867.

Larsen, D.B., & Milano, M.A.G. (1995). Are religion and spirituality clinically relevant in health care? *Mind-Body Medicine, 1,* 147–157.

Lewith, G., Kenyon, J., & Lewis, P. (1996). *Complementary medicine: An integrated approach.* New York: Oxford University Press.

Marwick, C. (1995). Should physicians prescribe prayer for health? Spiritual aspects of well-being considered. *JAMA, 273,* 1561–1562.

Meyer, T., & Mark, M. (1995). Effects of psychosocial interventions with adult cancer patients: A meta-analysis of randomized experiments. *Health Psychology, 14,* 101–108.

Montbriand, M.J. (1993). Freedom of choice: An issue concerning alternative therapies chosen by patients with cancer. *Oncology Nursing Forum, 20,* 1195–1201.

Montbriand, M.J. (1994). An overview of alternate therapies chosen by patients with cancer. *Oncology Nursing Forum, 21,* 1547–1554.

Morgan, B. (1989). *Growing together*. Pittsburgh: Pittsburgh Civic Garden Center.

Murphy, G.P., Morris, L.B., & Lange, D. (1997). *Informed decisions: The complete book of cancer diagnosis, treatment and recovery*. New York: Viking.

Nokes, K.M., Kendrew, J., & Longo, M. (1995). Alternative/complementary therapies used by persons with HIV disease. *Journal of the Association of Nurses in AIDS Care, 6*(4), 19–24.

Nurse's handbook of alternative and complementary therapies. (1999). Springhouse, PA: Springhouse Corp.

Pelton, R., & Overholser, L. (1994). *Alternatives in cancer therapy*. New York: Fireside.

Phalen, K.F. (1998). *Integrative medicine: Achieving wellness through the best of Eastern and Western medical practices*. Boston: Journey Editions.

Pilisuk, M., Wentzel, P., Barry, O., & Tennant, J. (1997). Participant assessment of a nonmedical breast cancer support group. *Alternative Therapy in Health and Medicine, 3*(5), 72–80.

Pimentel, E.S. (1998). Social images of the pain: From breast cancer patients. *Proceedings of the 17th International Cancer Congress* (p. 206). Geneva, Switzerland: International Union Against Cancer.

Rancour, P. (1994). Interactive guided imagery with oncology patients: A case illustration. *Journal of Holistic Nursing, 12*(2), 148–154.

Richardson, M.A., Post-White, J., Grimm, E.A., Moye, L.A., Singletory, S.E., & Justice, B. (1997). Coping, life attitudes, and immune response to imagery and group support after breast cancer treatment. *Alternative Therapy in Health and Medicine, 3*(5), 62–70.

Ryder, B.G. (1997). *The Alpha book on cancer and living*. Alameda, CA: The Alpha Institute.

Segen, J.C. (1998). *Dictionary of alternative medicine*. Stamford, CT: Appleton & Lange.

Shealy, C.N. (Ed.). (1996). *The complete family guide to alternative medicine*. Rockport, MA: Element Books.

Simonton, O.C., Matthews-Simonton, S., & Sparks, T.F. (1980). Psychological intervention in the treatment of cancer. *Psychosomatics, 21*(3), 226–227, 231–233.

Sloman, R. (1995). Relaxation and the relief of cancer pain. *Nursing Clinics of North America, 30,* 697–709.

Sloman, R., Brown, P., Aldana, E., & Chee, E. (1994). The use of relaxation to promote comfort and pain relief in persons with advanced cancer. *Contemporary Nurse, 3*(1), 6–12.

Smith, D.J. (1998). Horticultural therapy: The garden benefits everyone. *Journal of Psychosocial Nursing, 36*(10), 14–21.

Spiegel, D., & Moore, R. (1997). Imagery and hypnosis in the treatment of cancer patients. *Oncology, 11,* 1179–1189.

Syrjala, K.L., Donaldson, G.W., Davis, M.W., Kippes, M.E., & Carr, J.E. (1995). Relaxation and imagery and cognitive-behavioral training reduce pain during cancer treatment: A controlled clinical trial. *Pain, 63*(2), 189–198.

Troesch, L.M., Rodehaver, B.C., Delaney, E.A., & Yates, B. (1993). The influence of guided imagery on chemotherapy-related nausea and vomiting. *Oncology Nursing Forum, 20,* 1179–1185.

Wallace, K.G. (1997). Analysis of recent literature concerning relaxation and imagery interventions for cancer pain. *Cancer Nursing, 20*(2), 79–87.

Woodham, A., & Peters, D. (1997). *Encyclopedia of healing therapies*. New York: DK Publishing.

Workshop on Alternative Medicine. (1994). *Alternative medicine: Expanding medical horizons* (N.I.H. Publication No. 94-066). Washington, DC: Office of Government Publications.

Chapter Two

Bioelectromagnetic Therapies

Georgia M. Decker, MS, RN, CS-ANP, AOCN

Introduction

The study of bioelectromagnetic therapies gained recognition when German oncologist Ferdinand Sauerbruck raised awareness of low-frequency electromagnetic currents in the earth (geopathic zones). The theory of geopathic zones was based upon the belief that these low-frequency currents draw energy from humans' bodies, resulting in an increased risk of cancer and other diseases. This led to the studies that raised the issue of extremely low frequencies as a potential cause of cancer. Sauerbruck proposed that these low-frequency electrical currents could draw energy from the body and thereby increase the risk of developing cancer. In the 1960s, Ernst Hartmann continued to develop this theory (Willner, 1994). Recently, many studies have been conducted regarding the relationship between cancer incidence and exposure to high tension wires and electric appliances; it is believed that these exposures reduce the ability of the immune system to defend against infection and genetic change (Willner).

The amount and duration of exposure of these frequencies has been considered. Some studies refer to exposure to sunlight and acknowledge the affect that this can have on an individual's emotional and physical states. Those who consider this to be an important aspect of health and wellness would also be quick to point out that there is greater incidence of melancholia and depression during winter months when there is a decrease in exposure to light—seasonal affective disorder (SAD). These beliefs provide a basis for theories of health restoration and disease prevention (Willner, 1994).

Electromagnetic Field Therapy

Electrical currents can produce a variety of effects, including light spectrums and the conversion of electricity into magnetic fields. It is believed that a specific vibration can selectively destroy an abnormal cell while preserving normal cells (Willner, 1994). This theory is based on the belief that because all substances have a positive or negative charge, selective treatments would restore the balance of charges where there is an imbalance by neutralizing harmful charges. Knowledge about electromagnetic field therapy is limited because research in this area has been lacking.

Special Considerations

Electromagnetic field therapy is a type of energetic medicine that is based upon the theory of making corrections in human energy fields (Bock & Sabin, 1997). Research considerations include the concept that these human energy fields are under the influence of the destructive effects of environmental electromagnetism as electricity, microwaves, and nuclear radiation. Insufficient information is available to evaluate the potential carcinogenic effects of electromagnetic fields (Willner, 1994).

Cymatics/Aquasonics

Cymatics is a therapy that was born out of the theory that every living thing has its own particular magnetic field. Its name is derived from the Greek word *kyma,* which means "a great wave" (Bradford, 1996). Swiss scientist Hans Jenny pioneered research into the concept of using sound to influence magnetic fields, and British physician and osteopath Peter Manners continued research into this field and developed it into a therapy (Bradford). Practitioners of cymatic therapy use a special instrument that generates a frequency that is believed to be identical to healthy cells (Bradford). This instrument is pointed toward the area of the body that is causing symptoms to create corrective sound waves (see Figure 1). Depending on the treatment to be applied and the part of the body involved, the client will be asked to lie or sit on a specially designed structure. This therapy may be used in conjunction with acupuncture or osteopathy. It is not a cure for any disease.

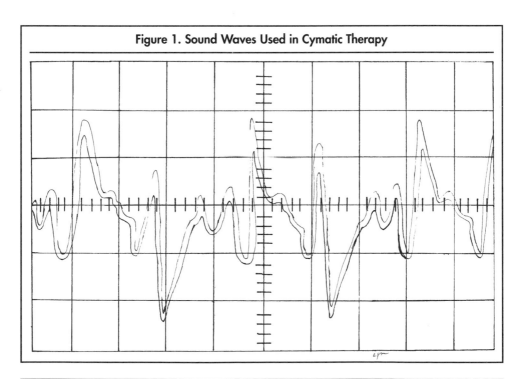

Figure 1. Sound Waves Used in Cymatic Therapy

Aquasonics is a form of cymatics that takes place in a heated pool. Sound waves alter the molecular structure of the water, which is believed to correct the frequency of the ailing part of the body. This form of therapy is preferred for people with mobility problems such as arthritis and physical disabilities (Bradford, 1996).

Special Considerations

Cymatic therapy is noninvasive and is considered to be safe for everyone when administered by a qualified practitioner. Although some question the therapeutic benefit of this therapy, no adverse effects have been recorded.

Magnet Therapy

Magnet energy as a cause of and potential cure for disease has fascinated healthcare professionals and others for many years (Rosenfeld, 1996). Some scientists believe that magnetism and electricity already are closely related and, together as electromagnetism, constitute a primary force in the universe. It is also believed that the various energy processes in the body generate their own magnetic fields, and manipulation of these fields has therapeutic potential (Gordon, 1996; Rosenfeld, 1996). Wolfgang Ludwig, director of the Institute for Biophysics in Horb, Germany, has written that magnetic field therapy has the potential to penetrate the human body and treat every organ. He believes that magnetic therapy has a wide range of indications without toxic side effects (Rosenfeld). Members of the scientific community, however, are somewhat reluctant to recognize the potential therapeutic benefits of magnets.

Two types of magnets exist—electromagnets and permanent magnets. Electrical currents flowing through cylindrical wire produce electromagnets. Their magnetic field of permanent magnets is created by the motion of electrons in the atoms of the magnetic material, usually iron or nickel. Once magnetized, the object maintains its magnetism. Magnetic fields from permanent magnets are always static, but this does not apply to electromagnets. However, similar therapeutic mechanisms are involved, and both have indications for use in contemporary medicine (Whitaker & Adderly, 1998). Permanent magnets cannot "pulse" their magnetism (i.e., turn it off and on at will). Electromagnetism is considered to be more powerful than permanent magnets. The strength of the magnetic field is measured as gauss, which represents the number of lines of magnetic force passing through one square centimeter. For example, a refrigerator magnet is about 200 gauss. Proponents of the use of magnets report therapeutic improvement in orthopedic injury, neuromuscular disease, and menstrual pain (Whitaker & Adderly).

Combining magnets with the tenets and points of acupuncture has become an area of interest among some practitioners. The therapeutic recommendation is that magnets be placed directly on the site of the discomfort. If that does not bring about relief, the magnets can be placed over the corresponding acupuncture points. In some cases, the use of magnets is recommended between acupuncture treatments to enhance their therapeutic benefit (Jacobs, 1996). This therapy requires the coordination of an appropriately trained healthcare professional. Magnetic therapy is considered by some to be effective when incorporated as a part of lifestyle changes, including nutrition, exercise, and stress management.

Special Considerations

Interest in this modality as a complementary/adjunctive therapy is growing. Caution, however, should be exercised when exploring this option, as the potential exists to hurt rather than help. Coordination of this therapy with the help of an appropriately trained practitioner of magnetic therapy is strongly recommended.

Pulsed Electromagnetic Energy (PEME)

The special apparatus used to deliver this therapy has recent U.S. Food and Drug Administration approval and has shown promise in the promotion of healing of bone fractures and reduction of soft-tissue inflammation. It has been used as a complementary therapy to enhance immune function, as well. Progress in research has diminished since the initial studies were completed (Willner, 1994).

Special Considerations

The qualifications of the practitioner are primary for safe administration and application of this therapy.

Transcutaneous Electrical Nerve Stimulation (TENS)

This therapy commonly is seen in the treatment of pain syndromes. It also has been successfully used in neuromuscular disorders. Therapy with TENS is an example of an "alternative" therapy that has become conventional and accepted. Wide variation exists in the results obtained utilizing this therapy. For some, this variation is a result of the electrodes being placed at the site of the pain rather than at the site of the origin of the pain.

Special Considerations

As a complementary therapy, TENS is considered best used when the practitioner is knowledgeable about and utilizes acupuncture points for electrode placement. Alternating currents comprise the stimulation component.

Acupuncture

Chinese health providers have used acupuncture for 5,000 years (Bradford, 1996). Jesuit missionaries returning from China in the 17th century are credited with reporting the therapeutic use of needles and coined the term *acupuncture* from the Latin *acus* (needle) and *punctura* (puncture or pricking). Chapter 3, "Alternative Systems of Medical Practice," discusses the historical perspective and foundation of acupuncture as an alternative/complementary therapy.

Acupuncture Procedure

Acupuncture utilizes steel needles with a length range from one-half inch to four inches and 26–36 gauge. Japanese acupuncture needles are thinner than traditional Chinese needles, and the needling techniques are considered to be more gentle (Collinge, 1996). Peterson (1996) reported that while most modern acupuncturists use disposable needles, some practitioners continue to employ reusable needles. Sterilization then becomes a concern, as cases of hepatitis B transmission through reusable needles have been reported ("Hepatitis B," 1992).

Selection of acupuncture needle insertion points is based upon assessment of the pulses and the five elements (see Chapter 3). Meridians provide additional information in the identification of the acupuncture points. Twelve main meridians (six yin and six yang) and many more minor ones form the energy channels throughout the body. Needles are inserted and advanced until the patient feels a tingling or numbness. The needles may be left in place, twisted, or connected to an electrical pulse generator (electroacupuncture). When left in place or twisted, the acupuncture needles remain in the patient's skin for up to 15 minutes (Collinge, 1996).

Simply stated, traditional practitioners attribute the positive effects of acupuncture to the restoration of yin-yang balance and the flow of ch'i (life force) (Bradford, 1997; Jacobs, 1996; Rosenfeld, 1996). Western scientists offer an alternative explanation—they believe that when the acupuncture point is stimulated by the placement of a needle, the body releases endorphins. Support for this theory is based on an experiment in which laboratory animals were given naloxone (an endorphin-blocking chemical) and then acupuncture; they exhibited no response to acupuncture (Rosenfeld).

Baischer (1995) conducted an uncontrolled study of the efficacy of acupuncture in 26 patients who suffered from chronic migraine headaches. Improvement of symptoms was noted in 18 patients, and 50% of patients reported a reduction in drug use for control of symptoms. Carlsson and Sjolund (1994) conducted a study of acupuncture and chronic pain in which 202 patients with pain—classified as nociceptive, neurogenic, or psychogenic—were treated with needle acupuncture (manual and electrical stimulation). The researchers concluded that a small segment of patients with nociceptive pain can expect pain relief for six months or longer after a treatment period of acupuncture.

Conflicting opinions exist regarding the effect of acupuncture in the treatment of substance abuse (McLellan, Grossman, Blaine, & Haverkos, 1993), primarily because the existing studies have involved small numbers of patients. Acupuncture has been used in general dentistry (Rosted, 1996) and has been used as an intervention to reduce postoperative oral surgery pain (Lao, Bergman, Langenberg, Wong, & Berman, 1995). Acupuncture practitioners also utilize points on the ear, which is known as auriculotherapy.

Special Considerations

The safety and efficacy of acupuncture are dependent upon the level of skill and training of the practitioner. Appropriate education and training are crucial. The issue of disposable versus reusable needles should be discussed prior to the initiation of treatment.

Electroacupuncture

Electroacupuncture is the use of electric current to stimulate acupuncture points. This therapy is based upon the premise that acupuncture points (the same as those used in traditional acupuncture) are of low electrical resonance. By stimulating the point with the use of direct current (as opposed to alternating current) administered through needles, the function of the organ is restored. Generally, electroacupuncture needles are left in place for a brief period of time, typically 30–60 seconds.

Special Considerations

Special considerations are the same as for acupuncture, PEME, and TENS.

Laser Acupuncture

Acupuncture using small, low-power lasers can be performed on clients who have a fear of needles. Laser acupuncture involves applying the laser beam to acupuncture points to stimulate energy flow. The lasers are said to be nondamaging to the skin, but the consistency of the equipment used has not been determined.

Special Considerations

Safety is dependent upon the level of experience of the acupuncturist with laser procedures and also on the equipment used.

Auriculotherapy

Auriculotherapy is the process of stimulating points on the outer ear (auricle) to affect corresponding areas of the body (see Figure 2). The ear is believed to mirror the shape of a fetus in the womb, with the earlobe representing the fetus' head. By superimposing the shape of the fetus onto the ear and stimulating the desired points, the corresponding parts of the body can be treated. Opinions differ as to the number of acupuncture points on the ear, ranging from 200 to more than 300. Auriculotherapy primarily is used for pain management in terminal illness and for the pain associated with labor and delivery (Bradford, 1997). It also has been used for treating substance abuse, allergies, and some respiratory disorders.

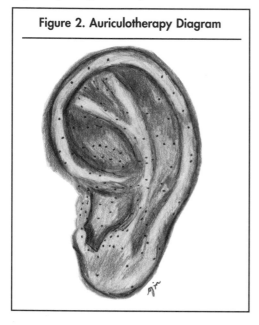

Figure 2. Auriculotherapy Diagram

Special Considerations

The safety and efficacy is dependent upon the practice of a qualified practitioner. The use of disposable needles and the proper disposal of used needles is imperative.

Hyperthermia

Recognition of the role of fever in healing has led to theories and research that includes stimulation of fever-like conditions as a treatment for a variety of conditions, which is known as hyperthermia (Rosenfeld, 1996). Fever is the body's defense against bacteria and viruses, and it also stimulates the production of antibodies and interferon. Healthcare providers sometimes try to mimic this response by using heat as therapy.

Heat also is used as local therapy—by applying heat to a small area of the body, as a regional therapy, by applying heat to a larger area or region, and even by drawing a person's blood, warming it to a specific temperature, and then reinfusing the warmed blood (Bock & Sabin, 1997). Some complementary practitioners believe that standing in hot water up to the neck every day for six months will relieve symptoms associated with chronic fatigue syndrome (Rosenfeld, 1996). In addition, Willner (1994) asserted that inducing hyperthermia may help to reduce the viral load in HIV infection and some cancers and that it also may have implications for Lyme disease.

Special Considerations

Hyperthermia must be administered very carefully, especially in the very young and the elderly. Because heat is a powerful vasodilator, special care must be taken with individuals with high or low blood pressure or multiple sclerosis and in pregnant women (Rosenfeld, 1996). Some practitioners may use *contrast hydrotherapy*. This entails alternating the application of hot and cold. The heat dilates blood vessels, and the cold then constricts them. The belief is that this sequencing will stimulate the circulatory system and relieve muscle spasms. Some holistic practitioners believe it may increase resistance to disease (Rosenfeld). Hyperthermia is being studied as both a single therapy and as a complementary or adjunctive therapy. It is being evaluated in conjunction with phototherapy as a cancer therapy (Willner, 1994). Scientific data, however, are not yet available.

Phototherapy/Light Therapy

Phototherapy has its foundation in psychiatric medicine and the diagnosis of SAD. Scientific medicine did not recognize the connection between mental health/mental illness and light/lack of light until the 1980s. However, Deepak Chopra has pointed out that in Ayurvedic medicine, light was used to treat a variety of illnesses in the sixth century B.C. (Rosenfeld, 1996). While no scientific evidence exists to support the claim that light improves other maladies, research exists to support the use of light boxes to treat SAD (Cassileth, 1998). One theory behind this is that light suppresses the overproduction of melatonin—an excess of melatonin can cause fatigue (Rosenfeld). Bright light therapy uses white light, which differs from color therapy. It is believed that these therapies share some common mechanisms. Bright light has the potential to cause damage to the eye.

Special Considerations

The research on the use of bright light therapy excluded patients with progressive retinal disease as a precautionary measure. Patients who are taking medications that increase photosensitivity should be monitored carefully. Many therapeutic light products are commercially available, but research has shown that a high-intensity fluorescent lamp that delivers 10,000-lux illumination is all that is needed. Caution should be taken to screen out ultraviolet light.

The therapeutic dose is 15 minutes to three hours daily. One *should not* look directly into the light and should sit under the light so that the illumination falls onto whatever one is reading or doing. Phototherapy is not a substitute for antidepressant therapy. Individuals who are interested in this therapy should seek the guidance of an appropriate healthcare professional (Rosenfeld, 1996).

Color Therapy

Belief in the healing effects of color dates back to ancient Egypt, India, and China. In Heliopolis, the ancient ruined city north of Cairo, rooms were designed to allow the sun's rays to break into the seven colors of the healing spectrum: red, orange, yellow, green, blue, indigo, and violet (Jacobs, 1996). These colors correspond to the body's seven chakras, which are centers of energy located along the axis of the spine. Contemporary thought has added magenta and turquoise to the spectrum and recognized the eighth chakra (see Figure 3).

The word *aura* has gained usage in contemporary discourse (e.g., "She has a certain aura."). In color therapy, *aura* refers to layers of color, the sum of which create a unique energy field for each individual. A healthy body's auric field is comprised of colors that complement one another and are in balance with one another. Treatment is aimed at bringing body energies into balance. Color therapy uses a variety of approaches for diagnosis and treatment. Some practitioners read one's aura to observe for color "balance." That is, because we seek balance, when one color is noted or used as therapy, its complement color also must occur or must be applied. It may involve the colors in one's home or workplace, as well as colors of clothing and food.

Figure 3. The Chakras

The chakras are recognized as components of the human energy system. Historically, seven chakras have been recognized, but an eighth has been added:

Base of spine	→ Red	Thymus	→ Turquoise
Sacrum	→ Orange	Throat	→ Blue
Solar plexus	→ Yellow	Brows	→ Violet
Heart	→ Green	Crown	→ Magenta

Special Considerations

Color therapy currently is being used as a complementary therapy in the treatment of psychological and physical illness. This therapy is believed to work well in conjunction with acupressure, acupuncture, and herbal therapy (Jacobs, 1996). Proponents believe that colored light is a powerful intervention and that color therapy must be performed by a specially trained practitioner who also will provide guidance in activities that can be accomplished at home, between sessions, to promote healing and restore balance. When considering color therapy, one should evaluate the color therapist to be sure that he or she is "seeing" with an open mind and heart. A practitioner's own condition can influence interpretation.

Polarity Therapy

Contemporary polarity therapy has enjoyed increased recognition, primarily through the leadership and influence of the American Polarity Therapy Association (APTA). They have established Standards for Practice that provide the basis of educational preparation and certification by APTA (Jacobs, 1996).

Polarity therapy is the science of balancing opposing energies (i.e., positive and negative) within the body. It is based in energy field theory and electromagnetic therapy and incorporates elements of manual healing methods. In this therapy, energy is seen as electromagnetic. Energy flow is believed to be governed by chakras, which control the energy needed for a specific body part to promote physical and emotional health. Each chakra and its corresponding body part are under the control of the five elements: ether, air, fire, water, and earth. It is a comprehensive therapy that involves the four dimensions of human experience: spirit, mind, feelings, and body. Good health means balance in and between dimensions. Polarity therapy is best known for its bodywork component; its basic premise is that touch affects the human energy field. The body is viewed as a magnet, with a positive charge at the top and a negative charge at the bottom. The hands each have a charge: postive on the right and negative on the left. Appropriate placement of the hands on the body can, therefore, have a stimulating or sedating effect based on knowing the major flow patterns and key intersections of the human energy field. Healing is considered to come from within the client. The practitioner is a facilitator (Jacobs, 1996).

Polarity therapy incorporates a vegetarian diet, movement and posture, and spiritual development. It does not focus on relieving symptoms as they are viewed as the body's attempt to heal itself; rather, it is viewed as aiding in healing by release of blocked or trapped energy and requires the participation of the client. Suggested indications for use include allergic, respiratory, digestive, and cardiovascular conditions and back pain. Stress-related illnesses are reported as responding positively to this therapy (Jacobs, 1996). Some view polarity therapy as soothing massage and see its benefits within that framework (Rosenfeld, 1996).

Special Considerations

Polarity therapy is not a cure for any condition but, under the guidance of a qualified practitioner, is considered to be safe. As with other bodywork therapies, it may promote a feeling of well-being.

Summary

"Over the years, scientists, pseudoscientists, and interested lay persons have been fascinated by the idea that magnetic energy may cause disease—and may also cure it" (Rosenfeld, 1996, p. 257). We know the body possesses its own magnetic fields and that these are now measurable. For example, we know that the brain emits electrical current. We also know that healing of bone fractures can be accelerated with magnetotherapy. There is much we do not know, as well. As this body of knowledge grows, we will be better able to distinguish those therapies that offer the most therapeutic value.

The credentials and training of the practitioner provide critical information for decision making. The risk-to-benefit ratio must be assessed and evaluated before participating in any of these therapies. We, as individuals, must assume final responsibility for our health and well-being.

References

Baischer, W. (1995). Acupuncture in migraine: Long-term outcome predicting factors. *Headache, 35,* 472–474.

Bradford, M. (Ed.). (1997). *Alternative healthcare.* San Diego: Thunderbay Press.

Carlsson, C.P., & Sjolund, B.H. (1994). Acupuncture and subtypes of chronic pain: Assessment of long-term results. *Clinical Journal of Pain, 10,* 290–295.

Cassileth, B.R. (1998). *The alternative medicine handbook: The complete reference guide to alternative and complementary therapies.* New York: Norton.

Collinge, W. (1996). *The American Holistic Association complete guide to alternative medicine.* New York: Warner Books Inc.

Fugh-Berman, A. (1997). *Alternative medicine: What works.* Baltimore: Williams & Wilkins.

Gordon, J.S. (1996). *Manifesto for a new medicine: Your guide to healing partnerships and the use of alternative therapies.* Reading, MA: Addison-Wesley.

Hepatitis B associated with an acupuncture clinic. (1992, November 27). *Communicable Disease Report. CDR Weekly, 2*(48), 219.

Jacobs, J. (1996). *The encyclopedia of alternative medicine.* Boston: Carlton Books Ltd.

Lao, L., Bergman, S., Langenberg, P., Wong, R.H., & Berman, B. (1995). Efficacy of Chinese acupuncture on postoperative oral surgery pain. *Oral Surgery, Oral Medicine, Oral Pathology, Oral Radiology, and Endodontics, 79,* 423–428.

McLellan, A.T., Grossman, D.S., Blaine, J.D., & Haverkos, H.W. (1993). Acupuncture treatment for drug abuse: A technical review. *Journal of Substance Abuse and Treatment, 10,* 569–576.

Peterson, J.R. (1996) Acupuncture in the 1990s. A review for the primary care physician. *Archives of Family Medicine, 5,* 237–240.

Rosenfeld, I. (1996). *Dr. Rosenfeld's guide to alternative medicine.* New York: Random House.

Rosted, P. (1996). The use of acupuncture in dentistry. *Australian Dental Journal, 41*(1), 61.

Whitaker, J.M., & Adderly, B.D. (1998). *The pain relief breakthrough: The power of magnets to relieve backaches, arthritis pain, menstrual cramps, carpal tunnel syndrome, sports injuries, and more.* Boston: Little, Brown & Co.

Willner, R. (1994). *The cancer solution.* Boca Raton, FL: Peltec Publishing Co., Inc.

Chapter Three

Alternative Systems of Medical Practice

Lisa Schulmeister, MN, RN, CS, OCN®

Introduction

Many patients are exploring alternative systems of medical practice because of their dissatisfaction with the existing healthcare system. Some seek unconventional therapy because of their desire to be cared for in a holistic manner. Others note the apparent health and longevity of certain cultural groups, such as the Amish, and adopt their daily practices or use their folk remedies. Several diverse alternative systems of medical practice have been identified—including naturopathy, homeopathy, environmental medicine, and folk medicine—each with its own unique history, beliefs, and practices. Although there is a paucity of large, randomized, controlled trials evaluating the efficacy of these treatments, sufficient evidence exists to suggest that many of these therapies can produce objective as well as subjective benefits in selected groups of patients. In view of the increasing popularity of complementary medicine among patients and general practitioners, there is now an urgent need to conduct high-quality research to determine how, or whether, these therapies may be interwoven with the more orthodox treatments currently available (Lewith & Watkins, 1996).

Anthroposophically Extended Medicine

Anthroposophy is a worldwide spiritual movement based on the work of Rudolf Steiner (1861–1925), an Austrian-born philosopher, scientist, artist, and educator. The word *anthroposophy* is derived from Steiner's view that "humanity (ANTHROPOS) has the inherent wisdom (SOPHIA) to transform both itself and the world" (Steiner, 1923, p. 3). Steiner described anthroposophy as a science of the spirit and a path of knowledge that can lead the spiritual in the human being to the spiritual in the universe. Although anthroposophy embraces a spiritual view of the human being, its emphasis is on knowing, not faith.

Steiner is considered to be the father of biodynamic agriculture, an organic process based on anthroposophic principles (Anthroposophic Press, 1997). He also is credited with innovative and holistic approaches to medicine. In 1925, Steiner and the Dutch physician Ita Wegman coauthored a book on medical practice that incorporated anthroposophic principles. Based on a spiritual-scientific model of human individuality, Steiner sought to reorient medical treatment to encompass the spiritual depths of human existence (Health and Human Services Dept., 1992).

Anthroposophically extended medicine does not regard illness as a chance occurrence or mechanical breakdown but rather as something intimately connected to an individual's biography. Handled appropriately, it presents opportunities for the individual to achieve new balance and maturity. The patient is seen and treated holistically and is viewed as having a body, soul, and spirit (Anthroposophic Press, 1997).

Anthroposophic Treatment

Anthroposophic physicians augment conventional medicine using a three-part model for understanding an illness. One component is the "sense-nerve" system, which includes the nervous system and the brain organization that supports the mind and the thinking process. The second is the "rhythmic" system, which includes physical processes of a rhythmic or periodic nature (e.g., breathing) and supports the emotional or feeling processes. The third is the "metabolic-limb" system, which includes digestion, elimination, metabolism, and voluntary movement. Illness is considered to be a deviation from the harmonious internal balance of the functions of the bodily self and the spiritual self. In this approach, a person's physical makeup is seen as continually interacting with his or her soul (Health and Human Services Dept., 1992).

Anthroposophic medicine integrates conventional practices with new and alternative remedies, dietary and nutritional therapy, rhythmic massage, hydrotherapy, art therapy, and counseling. In addition, hundreds of uniquely formulated medicines are used. Approximately 85% are prepared by a multiple dilution and potentiation process, and the remaining 15% are prepared similarly to traditional herbal medicines. The preparation of medications seeks to match the "archetypal forces" in plants, animals, and minerals with disease processes in humans and to stimulate healing (Anthroposophic Press, 1997).

Special Considerations

Anthroposophic medicine builds on three preexisting movements and therapeutics: (a) natural medicine or naturopathy, which involves the use of material substances in nondegraded, nonchemically altered forms, (b) homeopathy, which involves treating illness and disease based on the "law of similars" using homeopathic medicines, and (c) modern scientific medicine. Steiner insisted that anthroposophically extended medicine be practiced only on the foundation of a Western medical training and credentials; thus, only licensed medical doctors could become anthroposophic physicians (Health and Human Services Dept., 1992).

Ayurveda

The body of Hindu literature pertaining to medicine and health is called Ayurveda, the science of long life. Ayurveda is a short form for two Sanskrit words: *ayu*, which means "life," and *veda,* meaning "knowledge of." More than 5,000 years ago, a group of holy men in India known as the Rishis compiled the spiritual texts called the *Vedas* (or books of wisdom). The *Atharva Veda* was the source book of instructions for treating illness and disease. Ayurveda is a science of physical healing, diet, herbs, and massage or bodywork. It originally was intended as a means to support the body so that spiritual development could be pursued unhindered by health concerns (Gerson, 1993; Verma, 1995).

Proponents of Ayurveda view it as a *way of life* and claim that it is the oldest system of natural healing on earth. Its methods are noninvasive, nontoxic, and heavily dependent on the individual's willingness to participate by using the power of "self" (Health and Human Services Dept., 1992). Ayurveda recently has received considerable attention in the United States, primarily because of books on the topic written by Scott Gerson, MD, Andrew Weil, MD, and Deepak Chopra, MD (Leland & Power, 1997). Chopra (1991) stated that "the purpose of Ayurveda is to tell us how our lives can be influenced, shaped, extended, and ultimately controlled without interference from sickness or old age. The guiding principle of Ayurveda is that the mind exerts the deepest influence on the body, and freedom from sickness depends on contacting our own awareness, bringing it into balance, and then extending that balance to the body" (p. 6).

The Five Elements

The foundation of Ayurveda is a concept of vital energy called *prana*. *Prana* is considered to be the primal energy that enlivens the body and mind (Collinge, 1996). At the heart of Ayurveda is the concept that all of existence is comprised of five basic elements or energies (Gerson, 1993):

*   *Akasha* (ether)
*   *Vayu* (air)
*   *Tejas* (fire)
*   *Jala* (water)
*   *Prthivi* (earth)

More than their literal meanings, these terms represent principles of action and interaction that guide and shape all that exists. According to Ayurvedic wisdom, at conception, each individual is endowed with a unique pattern of organization of the five elements. In the body, the five elements undergo a further step of organization into three broader elements known as the *doshas: vata* (space and air), *pitta* (fire and water), and *kapha* (earth and water). Collectively, the three *doshas* form the *tridosha* and are considered to be the constituents that govern physiologic and psychological functions (see Table 1). The unique pattern of *doshas* in each person is called the person's *prakriti;* each person's *prakriti* is diagnosed and described according to which *doshas* naturally predominate and which are least influential in the person's functioning. For example, some people have a *prakriti* in which there is a clear dominance of a single *dosha,* either *vata, pitta,* or *kapha,* while others may have a more complex *prakriti,* such as *vata-pitta* or *vata-pitta-kapha* (Collinge, 1996; Gerson, 1993; Verma, 1995).

In Ayurveda, health is a state of balance and harmony among all of the elements or *doshas* within the person and harmony between the person and his or her surroundings. The optimal state is one in which the person is living in accordance with his *prakriti* at conception. Illness is believed to occur when the person falls out of equilibrium with this inborn pattern. Imbalances in specific *doshas*, called *vikriti* (deviating from nature), can be caused by chronic stress, eating certain foods, inadequate rest, environmental toxins, repressed emotions, and other factors. The resulting state of dishar-

Table 1. Qualities and Functions of the Three *Doshas*		
Dosha	**Qualities**	**Functions**
Vata (space and air)	Moving Quick Light Dry Clear	Movement Nervous system activities Elimination Respiration
Pitta (fire and water)	Hot Sharp Penetrating Acidic Slightly oily	Heat and metabolism Digestion Perception
Kapha (earth and water)	Solid Heavy Oily Cold Sweet Soft Immobile	Structural Musculoskeletal

mony weakens the *agni*, the fire that governs metabolism, which lowers the body's resistance as toxins accumulate in the body. The toxins are believed to circulate throughout the body and eventually build up in certain areas, causing symptoms and ultimately disease (Collinge, 1996; Gerson, 1993; Verma, 1995).

Health Promotion Through Ayurveda

Ayurveda's first priority is disease prevention, health promotion, and enhancement. Health is said to exist when all three *doshas* are in perfect equilibrium; all the *dhatus* (tissues) of the body are functioning properly; the three waste products (i.e., urine, feces, and perspiration) are produced and eliminated in normal quantities; the channels of the body are unimpeded; the appetite is good; the five senses are functioning normally; and the body, mind, and consciousness are in harmony. In perfect equilibrium, the individual is able to experience bliss (Gerson, 1993).

Ayurveda stresses self-examination so that the individual can become more self-aware and adhere to a lifestyle that leads to wholesomeness of being. Self-examination also enables the individual to acquire a sensitivity for detecting minor, subjective symptoms of an ailment. Self-examination is accomplished by regularly checking the stool for color, odor, and consistency; examining the urine for color, quantity, and frequency; observing for excess or deficient sweating; observing breathing for smoothness; feeling the body temperature; examining the pulse's strength and rhythm; and examining the colors of the tongue and eyes (Verma, 1995).

Diagnosing Illness

The Ayurvedic practitioner looks at the complete individual, viewing the entire body, the mind, the spirit, and the environment. Information from these four realms is deemed to be relevant, along with overt symptoms that are present. A pulse diagnosis also is made. For men, the right arm is used and for women, the left. The practitioner locates the radial artery and determines which of three pulse types is present: a *kapha* type, which is slow and gliding and is symbolized by a swan; a *pitta* type, which is quick, forceful, and throbbing and is symbolized by a frog; or a *vata* type, which is the fastest, feels irregular, and may waver and is symbolized by a snake (Chopra, 1991). Information is gathered and interwoven, along with the person's other natural characteristics, until it forms the person's *prakriti* (the individual's unique constitutional type). The practitioner then determines patterns of imbalance. Ayurvedic medicine does not identify a specific illness or a specific cause but instead gives an integrated description of the whole individual in which imbalance, or disharmony, is identified (Gerson, 1993).

Diseases are classified into three types: *vata* (space and air), *pitta* (fire and water), and *kapha* (earth and water), according to the predominant way in which the disease presents itself. For example, a productive cough would indicate a predominantly *kapha* condition. All diseases manifest the *dosha* that produces them (see Figure 1). According to Ayurveda, when the *tridosha* becomes unbalanced, disease, in some form, will occur (Gerson, 1993).

Three factors are believed to lead to imbalance of the *doshas*. The first is misuse of the mind and body, which includes all thoughts or actions that breach the natural order of human life and cause impairment of the intellect, emotions, and

Figure 1. General Disease Categories of the *Tridosha*		
Vata (Space and air)	**Pitta** (Fire and water)	**Kapha** (Earth and water)
Nervous tissue	Fevers	Respiratory (asthma, influenza, etc.)
Tissue atrophy	Blood dyscrasias	Renal
Headaches	Hepatic	Sinusitis
Constipation	Hyperacidity	Edema
Arthritis	Skin	Tumors
Dryness	Inflammatory	Abnormal growths and secretion

memory. The second factor is unhealthy association of the sense organs with sense objects, which includes overstimulation and understimulation of the five sense organs. Influences of time and season comprise the third factor. Inappropriate use of the intellect, emotions, diet, lifestyle, sense organs, climate, and other factors are believed to create an imbalance of the *doshas*. This imbalance results in a diminished *agni* (biological fire), which leads to *ama* formation (incompletely digested food mass). *Ama* is believed to obstruct the proper flow of nutrients and accumulates in the body. The accumulation of *ama* results in the manifestation of disease. Ayurveda recognizes six stages in the course of a disease, which describe the disruption and evolution of the imbalanced *doshas* (Gerson, 1993):

1. Accumulation (*sancaya*)
2. Aggravation (*prakopa*)
3. Dispersion (*prasara*)
4. Relocation (*sthana samsraya*)
5. Manifestation (*vyakti*)
6. Maturation (*bheda*)

Collectively, the six stages are called *sata kriyakala,* which means "six-runged ladder." According to the movement of the imbalanced *doshas* through the body, three courses of disease have been identified in Ayurvedic medicine: internal, external, and middle. The internal course includes the digestive tract, the external includes the skin, and the middle includes tissues, bones, nerves, and organs (Gerson, 1993).

Ayurvedic Treatment

Ayurvedic medicine uses various methods for disease prevention and treatment. A goal of the Ayurvedic approach is to maintain health by harmonizing *doshas* with the environment. Minor imbalances can be treated quickly and easily if the individual frequently performs self-examination and identifies imbalances through early detection. A variety of measures also are used when disease states are more advanced and have "taken root in the physiology" (Gerson, 1993, p. 78).

Meditation

Meditation is the preeminent treatment in Ayurvedic medicine. Without meditation, proponents believe, the true healing potential of Ayurvedic medicine cannot be realized. Meditation is a technique that allows the mind to settle into a state of complete stillness while remaining awake. The ancient founders of Ayurveda noted that the most profound perceptions about the nature of man and reality came not through logic but from direct experience. Thus, the truths of Ayurveda are believed to be realized through intuition rather than through empirical sensory experience (Gerson, 1993; Lad, 1984).

Diet

A basic Ayurvedic principle is that health and well-being largely depend on how well the digestive system provides nutrition for the physical body. The digestive system plays a vital role in assimilation and elimination of nutrients. Ayurveda places great emphasis on the condition of the bowels and the interaction between the mind and the digestive system. According to Ayurvedic principles, nutrients should be chosen according to the season, the individual's constitution, and the specific *dosha* imbalances that are present. Other important dietary considerations include not eating until the previous meal is completely digested, not eating when nervous or angry, avoiding distractions while eating, chewing thoroughly, eating the largest meal at noon, and taking a 20-minute walk after dinner (Gerson, 1993).

Abhyanga (Self-Massage)

According to Ayurveda, recent and distant past lives can be observed in the present body structure—the chronicle of past experiences can be read in the individual's physical form. Individuals who have held their bodies in unnatural postures limit the free flow of *prana,* or vital energy. The ancient Ayurvedic sages discovered 107 points, known as *marma* points, distributed throughout the body through which *prana* must flow for health to be maintained. If the flow of *prana* through one or more *marma* points is disrupted, it is believed that disease will manifest (Gerson, 1993).

Self-massage, or *abhyanga,* is thought to unblock and balance the flow of *prana* through the *marma* points. Massage is performed with oils that are selected according to each individual's constitution and particular imbalance. Prior to beginning self-massage, the individual lies quietly and takes deep breaths while the oil is heated to a few degrees warmer than skin temperature. The particular self-massage technique is determined by the disorder being treated and by *doshic* predominance. Generally, self-massage is performed for 15–20 minutes daily by vigorously massaging certain body points in a circular motion. Self-massage usually is initiated in the palm of the hand or sole of the foot because these locations are believed to contain several *marma* points. Massage is thought to cleanse the body, eliminate toxins, open channels, and rejuvenate the mind and body (Gerson, 1993; Verma, 1995).

Herbal Therapies

The ancient Ayurvedists believed that consciousness permeated all forms of life. They felt that all of life is interconnected and integrated and represents a synergistic expression of mutual support and nourishment. Herbal plants were believed to contain energy and produce an enlivening effect on consciousness.

The entire panorama of Ayurvedic herbal medicine is vast. Proponents of Ayurveda recommend that qualified Ayurvedic practitioners be consulted to prescribe appropriate herbal therapy. The general principles guiding herbal therapy include using herbs that are indigenous to the patient's region, using mild herbs, and always using herbs in conjunction with meditation, diet, and other Ayurvedic approaches to health. Without the holistic support of other approaches, it is believed that very little benefit can be expected from herbal therapies (Gerson, 1993). Patients typically are advised to consume herbal therapies three times a day as an infusion (tea), decoction (boiling hard or woody substances), or powder. Some examples of Ayurvedic herbal remedies include (Gerson):

1. For acne: Make a poultice of one-half teaspoon each of sandalwood, turmeric, and myrrh powder mixed with sufficient aloe vera gel to make a paste; apply and leave on area for 30 minutes; rinse with warm water.
2. For depression: Make an infusion of St. John's wort, ginkgo biloba, ginseng root, and skullcap.
3. For laryngitis: Gargle with hot water and one teaspoon each of bayberry and red sage.

Dinacarya (Daily Routine)

Ayurveda places great emphasis on regularity in daily routine. By following a lifestyle that is in harmony with the natural cycle of the day, it is believed that strength, intelligence, and health will result. A daily routine that includes awakening at a consistent time, followed by exercising, nourishing the body, meditating, and self-massaging, is thought to promote harmony (Gerson, 1993).

Fasting

According to Ayurvedic practices, fasting one day a week is recommended for normal, healthy individuals. It is believed to be an effective initial treatment for many diseases because it rids the body of toxins and enlivens *agni*, the digestive fire. Many variations of fasting are described in Ayurveda, ranging from water fasts to fasts incorporating various juices, teas, and broths. Individuals with a high *kapha* constitution are thought to benefit from longer fasts, generally three to seven days in duration. *Before* undertaking a fast, it is recommended that an Ayurvedic practitioner be consulted (Gerson, 1993; Verma, 1995).

Aromatherapy

The essential oils of many plants are used in massage and steam inhalation or in aroma-diffuser pots to produce odors that have a therapeutic effect on the mind and body. In Ayurveda, aromas are used to pacify aggravated or imbalanced *doshas*. The method of application of aromatherapy is determined by the *prakriti* (constitutional type) of the individual being treated. *Vata* individuals are believed to respond best to massage techniques that incorporate aroma oils; *pitta* individuals are most responsive to aroma-pot therapy; and *kapha* types are believed to be best suited to steam-inhalation techniques (Gerson, 1993).

Other Ayurvedic Treatments

Ayurvedic practitioners frequently are trained in climatology, mineralogy, and psychology. Some also are trained in predictive astrology. Treatments used by some Ayurvedic practitioners include the use of color therapy, crystals, mantras, and gems. The healing power of gems and stones is believed to be activated by wearing them as ornaments or by placing them in water overnight and drinking the water the next day. For healing, amethysts, bloodstones, and pearls are recommended (Gerson, 1993; Lad, 1984).

Research on Efficacy of Ayurveda

Few randomized, controlled studies assessing the efficacy of Ayurvedic treatments have been conducted. In a study conducted by Paranjpe and Kulkarni (1995), 82 patients with acne vulgaris were randomized to receive one of four different Ayurvedic treatments or a placebo. A significant reduction in lesion count was observed in the group that received a salve containing the herb Sunder Vati; no significant differences were observed in the lesion counts of the other three treatment groups or the placebo group. All Ayurvedic treatments were reported to be well-tolerated.

Smit et al. (1995) empirically assessed 14 species of Ayurvedic herbal drugs with reported tumor-destroying abilities. Using the microculture tetrazolium (MTT) assay procedure, and using the parameter of a 50% growth inhibition to measure cytotoxicity, they found that the flowers of *Calotropis procera* and the nuts of *Semecarpus anacardium* displayed cytotoxic effects; the other plants did not. Prasad, Parry, and Chan (1993) evaluated the efficacy of Maharishi Amrit Kalash ambrosia (MAK-5) and Maharishi Amrit Kalash nectar (MAK-4) on murine and human melanoma cells in culture. MAK-4 inhibited growth of human melanoma cells, and murine melanoma cells were sensitive to MAK-5. Continuing research on the use of Ayurvedic herbs as a potential cancer treatment currently is being conducted.

Special Considerations

Panchakarma is the therapeutic means by which excess *doshic* energies are eliminated. *Panchakarma* means "the five actions," and these actions allude to the natural and gentle cleansing actions that normally occur in everyone. The first, *nasya*, refers to the administration of substances, such as ginger powder and powdered peppers, via the nasal passages to remove excess *kapha dosha* from the head and neck. *Vamana*, or vomiting therapy, is used to remove excess *kapha dosha* from the stomach and chest and usually is performed daily, first thing in the morning, on an empty stomach. It is believed that the lungs are cleaned when the stomach is cleaned because the stomach and lungs arise from the same primitive embryonal tissue. Methods of inducing vomiting include drinking herbal infusions of calamus, pennyroyal, or licorice, followed by rubbing the back of the tongue. *Virechana* involves the ingestion of an oleating substance followed by a gentle laxative to eliminate excess *pitta dosha* and cleanse the blood, liver, small intestine, and sweat glands. *Basti* involves the application of medicated oils and herbalized decoctions as an enema to remove excess *vata dosha* from the colon, rectum, lumbosacral region, and bones. The literal meaning of *basti* is "urinary bladder"; ancient Ayurvedists used the urinary bladders of cows and goats to administer the enemas. The substances used for *basti* vary widely and include castor and olive oils, herbal oils, and broths of meat and bone marrow. *Basti* is used as a treatment for lower-back pain, constipation, arthritis, and other conditions. *Raktamokshana* involves the removal of small quantities of blood from a vein to eliminate toxins and excess *pitta dosha* from the blood, lymph, and deeper tissues. *Because of its invasive nature, this therapy is used less commonly today than in the past, and it is recommended that this procedure should be administered only by a physician.* Bloodletting is thought to stimulate the immune system and is used to treat skin disorders, tumors, and jaundice (Gerson, 1993; Verma, 1995). Bloodletting is contraindicated in individuals who are experiencing anemia, edema, and weakness and is not recommended for the elderly or children (Lad, 1984).

A study of 29 people who had taken Ayurvedic metal-mineral tonics revealed that five had lead poisoning and required chelation therapy. A wide range of lead content was found in the Ayurvedic preparations taken (Prpic-Majic, Pizent, Jurasovic, Pongracic, & Restek-Samarzija, 1996). Bayly et al. (1995) reported a series of five cases of lead poisoning associated with Ayurvedic preparations. One patient also had high levels of mercury; another, arsenic; and a third, aluminum and tin. Other reports of mercury exposure and nodular reactions to oral mercury during Ayurvedic treatments have been reported (Jun, Min, Kim, Chung, & Lee, 1997; Wendroff, 1997). Dunbabin, Tallis, Popplewell, and Lee (1992) published a case report of a 37-year-old man who presented with abdominal pain following ingestion of Ayurvedic medicine. He was diagnosed with a low-grade hepatitis, normocytic anemia, and lead poisoning. His symptoms resolved following chelation therapy. Aconite, an Ayurvedic herbal remedy, was found to produce cardiotoxity in one patient (Gohel & Dave, 1991), and otitis externa and facial cellulitis was reported to occur in two patients using Ayurvedic ear cleaners (Berry & Collymore, 1993).

The rhizome of *Costus speciosus,* the tuber of *Nephrolepsis,* and the bulb of *Stephania hernandifolia* were found to produce a significant hypoglycemic effect in a study by Mosihuzzaman et al. (1994) and may become a future source of oral hypoglycemic agents. However, in nondiabetic individuals, these three plants may pose a health risk because of their ability to rapidly and dramatically drop serum glucose levels. The purification therapies pose serious health threats to compromised individuals and should not be self-administered.

Ayurvedic Practice

At the time of this printing, approximately 10 Ayurvedic clinics are operating in North America, and more than 200 physicians have received training as Ayurvedic practitioners through the American Association of Ayurvedic Medicine and have incorporated Ayurveda into their clinical practice. In India, Ayurvedic practitioners receive state-recognized training along with their physician counterparts in the state-supported systems for conventional Western biomedicine and homeopathic medicine. In addition, a number of these Indian-trained Ayurvedic physicians practice or teach Ayurveda in the United States (Health and Human Services Dept., 1992).

Cost of Ayurvedic Treatment

The cost of Ayurvedic consultations varies widely. An initial consultation may cost $40 to $100 or more, depending on the credentials of the practitioner and the length of the visit. Follow-up visits are less costly. Because few follow-up visits usually are required, Ayurveda tends to be relatively inexpensive in terms of professional services. The cost of herbs varies and may range from $10 to $50 or more each month. Herbs typically can be purchased directly from the practitioner. Insurance coverage generally is limited to licensed physicians who also incorporate Ayurveda into their regular clinical practice (Collinge, 1996).

Community-Based Healthcare Practices

An example of a community-based healthcare system is Alcoholics Anonymous (A.A.). Founded in 1935 by two alcoholics, Bob Smith, MD, and Bill Wilson, A.A. is a client-centered self-help fellowship that is considered to be the most successful method for supporting sobriety. In this treatment approach, alcoholism is viewed as a disease that is controllable only by the cessation of drinking. The concept of loss of control is a component of the A.A. philosophy, and members are required to comprehend the extent to which they have lost control of their lives as the first step in a 12-step program. Members attend group support meetings at least weekly, and meetings typically are offered daily at various times. According to estimates, A.A. has approximately a half-million members worldwide (Health and Human Services Dept., 1992).

Environmental Medicine

Environmental medicine is an alternative system of medical practice based on the science of assessing the impact of environmental factors on health. It includes the study of the interfaces among chemicals, foods, and inhalants in the environment and the biologic function of the individual (Moore, 1997). Diet and environment are estimated to play a role in approximately 90% of all cases of cancer and cardiovascular disease (U.S. Public Health Service, 1990).

Theron Randolph, MD, the father of environmental medicine, identified a wide range of medical problems in the 1940s that he believed were caused by food allergies. Using the method of identifying food allergies by avoiding the suspected food for at least four days before administering a food challenge, Randolph was able to identify food-related triggers for symptoms associated with arthritis, asthma, depression, anxiety, colitis, fatigue, and other disorders. In the 1950s, Rudolph noted that chemicals such as natural gas, industrial solvents, and automobile exhaust fumes were responsible for previously unrecognized health problems. Certain individuals were found to be more sensitive than others to exposure to these substances. Through careful, detailed, environmentally focused clinical observations, Randolph and others developed a new model and associated clinical principles, which involve assessing the interaction between the individual's internal state and exposure to external factors (Health and Human Services Dept., 1992).

Diagnosing Illness

The environmental medicine practitioner obtains a detailed chronological history to identify environmentally focused events and stressors over time. Extensive information is obtained about the home and work environment, and many questions are asked about exposure to potentially hazardous substances. The environmental medicine practitioner also obtains a thorough medical history and conducts an in-depth physical examination.

The factors contributing to the patient's degree of sensitivity are believed to be related to the patient's genetic makeup, nutritional status, detoxification abilities, and total allergic and chemical load. Biochemical individuality determines the adequacy of nutritional stores, influences the ability to operate the detoxification pathways effectively and, thus, contributes to the individual's degree of sensitivity. Other factors that can induce immune system dysfunction (e.g., emotional stress) are thought to have a major impact on the outcome of an exposure to a chemical toxin, a food, or an inhalant (Health and Human Services Dept., 1992).

The onset of illness coincides with the person's inability to continue coping with the total allergic load. Illness may occur as a result of a large, acute exposure, or as a result of chronic, low-level exposure to substances to which the person is sensitive. Environmental medicine practitioners believe that large amounts of toxic substances affect all of those exposed, but minute amounts affect only those who are susceptible to the material. Thus, a susceptible person may become ill from a small exposure, while one who is not susceptible experiences no ill effects (Brooks, Gochfeld, Herzstein, Schenker, & Jackson, 1995).

The course of events in environmental illnesses is explained by adaptation— the process by which the body attempts to maintain homeostasis. Four distinct phases of adaptation are thought to exist: (a) preadapted-nonadapted (alarm), (b) adapted (masked), (c) maladapted, and (d) exhausted-nonadapted (Health and Human Services Dept., 1992). The first three stages occur sequentially and, if left uninterrupted, can lead to the fourth stage, or the onset of disease.

Another observed event in environmental medicine is the spreading phenomenon, which is the development of a new susceptibility to previously tolerated substances or the spreading of susceptibility to new target organs. This phenomenon often is observed in individuals with pesticide exposure, which causes one to become reactive to many other chemicals. In the switch phenomenon, symptoms change and can affect different organ systems. This movement has been described as the bipolar and biphasic responses of biological mechanisms and includes stimulatory phases and withdrawal phases (Health and Human Services Dept., 1992).

The diagnostic process involves recognizing effects of total allergic load, the spreading phenomenon, the switch phenomenon, and biochemical individuality so that the etiology of the illness can be determined. The physical examination and laboratory studies assess for evidence of nutritional deficiencies, organ system dysfunction, and disorders of the detoxification systems. Testing for allergies and hypersensitivity also is conducted. Various techniques are used to test a wide range of antigens, such as bacteria, foods, chemicals, dust, mites, pollens, and molds (Brooks et al., 1995; Health and Human Services Dept., 1992).

Environmental Medicine Treatment

Environmental medicine treatment approaches require a thorough understanding of the nature of environmentally induced illness. Immunotherapy often is used to reduce sensitivity to environmental antigens. Patient education is an important component of treatment; emphasis is placed on reducing exposure to environmental hazards at home and work. Public education strategies involve informing groups about alternatives to the use of chemicals and other hazardous substances; for example, farmers are taught about alternatives to using chemicals as pesticides (Health and Human Services Dept., 1992).

When intoxication or poisoning by metals or related compounds occurs, the treatment is specific to the particular type of substance involved. Many substances have been found to cause ill effects (see Figure 2), and most induce both acute and chronic clinical

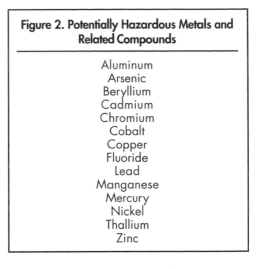

Figure 2. Potentially Hazardous Metals and Related Compounds

Aluminum
Arsenic
Beryllium
Cadmium
Chromium
Cobalt
Copper
Fluoride
Lead
Manganese
Mercury
Nickel
Thallium
Zinc

effects. Treatment varies and may include chelation therapy with dimercaprol for arsenic intoxication, use of topical steroid preparations to treat the toxic effects of chromium, or hemodialysis for mercury poisoning (Rosenstock & Cullen, 1994).

Dietary Management

Dietary management is based on avoidance of food antigens and on the four-day rotation diet. With the rotation diet and avoidance of repetitive food exposures, sensitivity to foods can be reduced in susceptible individuals (Rosenstock & Cullen, 1994). Nutritional supplements also are prescribed as indicated by objective nutritional assessment testing as well as symptomatology.

Research on Treatment Efficacy

Environmental medicine research has been directed at both clinical treatment of ill patients and evaluation of the diagnostic and treatment techniques used by environmental medicine practitioners. Support for environmental approaches has been documented in the treatment of arthritis, asthma, colitis, depression, eczema, allergies, migraines, and urticaria (Health and Human Services Dept., 1992).

Environmental Medicine Practice

Today, the nonoccupational environment rivals or exceeds the occupational environment as a source of health concerns among the public at large. Prominent environmental health issues include, but are not limited to, the following (Kilbourne, 1994):

- Exposure to lead in drinking water
- Exposure to radon in indoor air

- Exposure to halogenated organic compounds (e.g., dioxin)
- Effects of substances added to the foods of animals that produce milk and meat
- Effects of substances added to foods
- Hazardous waste disposal
- Water and air pollution
- Consequences of global warming and depletion of the stratospheric zone.

Special Considerations

Environmental medicine increasingly is being affiliated with occupational health and safety in many practice settings in the United States and Australia (Emmett, 1996). Environmental medicine has been called the corollary of occupational medicine, and 50% of medical residency programs in the United States and Canada offer occupational and environmental medicine training opportunities (Cordes, Rea, Rea, & Peate, 1996). National certification in occupational and environmental medicine also is offered in the United States (Cordes et al.).

Folk Medicine

Complex systems of health beliefs and practices exist across and within cultural groups. In addition, variations of cultural beliefs and practices are found across social class boundaries and even within family groups. In the United States, the most widely accepted healthcare system is the biomedical model. Despite its wide use, however, this model is thought by many to be culture-specific, culture-bound, value-laden, and representative of only one end of a continuum of health care. At the opposite end of the continuum is the traditional healthcare model, which espouses popular beliefs and practices that diverge from medical science. People who subscribe to the traditional model follow unique health beliefs and practices that are predominantly culturally influenced and historically preserved (Giger & Davidhizar, 1995).

Folk medicine represents an alternative system of medical practice that is steeped in tradition. It encompasses the traditional healthcare beliefs and practices that are handed down from one generation to the next and typically are categorized according to their cultural origin.

African American Folk Practices

The origins of African American folk practices can be traced back to West African practices that were brought to the United States and handed down from generation to generation. African American folk medicine took root not only as an offshoot of cultural heritage but also as a necessity when African Americans were denied access to the biomedical healthcare system. African American folk medicine currently is practiced in the South and some urban northern areas. Folk medicine practices, which are spirituality-based, use prayer and herbal remedies as the mainstays of treatment and may include witchcraft, magic, and voodoo practices (Campinha-Bacote, 1992, 1998; Cates, 1996; Cherry & Giger, 1995; Gustafson, 1989). The use of voodoo is not restricted to the African Americans with whom it originated; it also was adopted by the Creoles, a cultural group derived from French and Spanish origin, and continues to be practiced in some southern locations, such as New Orleans (Reed, 1990). Examples of voodoo treatments include wearing anklets made of garlic, drinking the milk from a cow that has just had its first calf, severing chicken heads and smearing the blood on the body, and using voodoo dolls.

The African American system of folk medicine perceives illness as either a natural or unnatural occurrence. Natural events are those that are in harmony with nature (e.g., sun shines, rain falls) and provide people who believe in and practice folk medicine with a certain degree of predictability in the events of daily living. Conversely, unnatural events (e.g., hurricanes, floods) represent disharmony with nature, which makes the events of day-to-day living unpredictable. Another aspect of this system is a belief in opposing forces (i.e., the belief that everything has an opposite). Health is believed to be a gift from God, and illness is viewed as punishment from God or a retribution for sin and evil (Snow, 1983).

African American folk medicine care typically is provided by an "old lady" or "granny" who serves as a local medical consultant and has extensive knowledge about many different home remedies (containing spices, herbs, and roots) that are used to treat common illnesses. A second type of practitioner is the "spiritualist," who combines spiritual beliefs, rituals, and herbal medicines to cure illnesses and ailments. A third type of practitioner is the voodoo priest or priestess (or queen) who uses voodoo, magic, and witchcraft to mobilize the forces of good and evil and dispel hexes or spells (Cherry & Giger, 1995).

Some African Americans choose to use folk medicine because of tradition. Others use folk practices because they lack access to primary medical care or because of discriminatory practices in health care and social policies that have occurred historically (Cherry & Giger, 1995).

Amish Folk Practices

The Amish movement began in 1525, and most of today's Amish are descendants of Jakob Ammann, a 17th century Mennonite leader who advocated strict community conformity (Quillin, 1996). Today, about 70,000 Amish reside in 50 communities in the United States and Canada (Quillin). Amish folk medicine is practiced by the Amish themselves, as well as by a growing number of non-Amish people who have taken notice of the long, healthy lives typically led by the Amish. The Amish use folk medicine almost exclusively; professional care is only sought for very high fevers, when surgery or stitches are needed, or when there is a need to be hospitalized (Wenger, 1995).

The Amish maintain that health and happiness only are attainable when humans are in harmony with the laws of God and nature. Ancient biblical recommendations are incorporated into their everyday lifestyle and include hard work, respect for others, kindness, simplicity, the importance of family, and resourcefulness. Rejection of worldliness and materialism is a central belief (Buccalo, 1997; Quillin, 1996; Yoder, 1997). Good health is considered to be a gift from God, and the Amish believe that their longevity is a reward for their hard work and "clean living." The Amish use a wide variety of folk healthcare providers, including reflexologists, herbalists, lay midwives for home births, and *brauche* practitioners. *Brauche* is a practice of physical manipulations similar to therapeutic touch in which a person with the gift of healing places his or her hands near the patient's head or abdomen to draw illness from the body (Brewer & Bonalumi, 1995).

The Amish have clung to their traditional practices and have shunned many modern medical practices that are considered routine, such as childhood immunizations. However, an outbreak of polio in the Amish community in 1979 left more parents willing to immunize their children (Brewer & Bonalumi, 1995).

The Amish use several therapies to maintain or restore good health, including the following (Quillin, 1996):

- Solar therapy: The Amish work outside as much as possible and are advocates of "natural light." They also eat fresh foods that contain "light energy." They believe that "light energy" is lost when chemical fertilizers are used and food is commercially processed.
- Herbal and natural therapies: The world's "greatest pharmacy" is believed to lie in the humble plants scattered throughout the planet. Herbal remedies are used to treat a wide variety of disorders, ranging from diaper rash (apply cornstarch) to diarrhea (drink tea made from slippery elm and eat rice).
- Physiotherapy: Exercise and body maintenance are believed to be crucial in maintaining healthy muscles, bones, and circulatory powers.
- Diet therapy: Proper digestion, elimination, and absorption are viewed as crucial for health.
- Respiratory therapy: Breathing fresh, clean, unpolluted air is thought to bring oxygen to the cells. Homes should be clean and well-ventilated, and aromatic herbs are used to improve breathing.

- Hydrotherapy: Water is viewed as the "river of life" in the body. Water is used inside and outside the body.
- Spiritual therapy: Emotional illness is thought to bring on physical illness. Components of spiritual therapy include love, alms, blessings, honoring the Sabbath, and celebrating holidays.

Appalachian Folk Practices

Approximately 20.7 million people live in the federally defined Appalachian regions spanning 400 counties in 13 states; most live in rural, nonfarming areas with high rates of poverty (U.S. Department of Commerce, Bureau of Census, 1993). While some Appalachians obtain professional medical care, many continue to use folk medicine to treat a number of diseases.

Appalachians generally believe that life is controlled by nature and that sickness is the will of God. Disability is viewed as inevitable because it is believed to accompany aging (Purnell & Counts, 1998). Because they believe in an external locus of control, most Appalachians avoid hospitals and fear hospitalization because it is associated with death (Small, 1995).

Special Considerations

In the Appalachian folk system, folk healers commonly are called "granny women" or "herb doctors." Folk healers are accepted and respected because they are familiar with the culture, are mountain people themselves, and can be trusted. Folk healers use a variety of herbs, poultices, and tonics to treat an array of illnesses (Small, 1995). A tradition of using unorthodox treatments for cancer exists in the Appalachian south (Cavender, 1996).

While many Appalachians seek professional care when they become very ill, they first turn to the folk medicine system. Factors that influence the use of folk practitioners include the lack of access to conventional healthcare facilities as a result of rugged terrain, the economic conditions, and a shortage of community-based healthcare providers (Purnell & Counts, 1998).

Cajun Folk Practices

During the 1760s, the Cajuns—French refugees going to Louisiana from the maritime provinces of Canada's east coast—brought their own brand of natural healing, a blend of home recipes developed in the provinces of New Brunswick and Nova Scotia and traditional remedies that they brought from France. Settling in the rural southwest bayou area, most Cajuns became fishermen or farmers (Ancelet, 1994). During decades of oppression and exile, the early Cajuns survived through careful use of scarce resources. Although modern society offers technological advances, this close-knit group of hearty individuals frequently chooses to leave many traditional practices unchanged (Oriol, 1995).

Cajun folk medicine is a combination of herbal medicine and belief in supernatural healing powers. When the Cajuns first settled in Louisiana, a granny midwife was summoned whenever someone became ill or was injured. The granny midwife's role in the community extended well beyond assisting women in the birthing process; she also could treat a wide variety of ailments. Grannies often used plant-derived substances in their treatments and employed simple treatment measures, such as using burlap to bind a broken leg to a tree branch to immobilize it and facilitate healing. As explorers passed through Louisiana on their way to Texas, they introduced other folk healing methods, namely supernatural healing. Subsequently, three separate and distinct types of practitioners provided care: (a) the *remedeman*, a dispenser of herbal medicine, domestic remedies, and patent medicines available without prescription, (b) the faith healer, called *traiteurs* ("treaters"), who heal by saying prayers, using charms, performing religious chants and incantations, and the laying on of hands (considered to be white magic), and (c) the "hoodoo-men," who practice black magic (*gris-gris*, a French word for magic charm, hex, or spell) and are believed to be able to both cause and cure diseases and illnesses (Reed, 1990).

For Cajuns who continue to cling to a traditional lifestyle, the concept of health equals the absence of disease. Happiness is conceptualized as "being well and having enough to eat" and is said to occur when "the neighbor's wife dies instead of yours" (Touchstone, 1983, p. 21).

Special Considerations

Cajun folk medicine treatment largely is based on the use of herbs as medication. The herbs are prepared by a variety of processes, including infusions (steeping), decoctions (simmering in boiling water), tinctures (adding herbs to water or ethyl alcohol), plasters, poultices, powders, and salves. The blackberry (*Rubus louisianus*), considered the wonder herb of the backwoods, is used in more ways than any other herb. Blackberry roots are used in the treatment of diarrhea, sore throat, swelling of the limbs, and skin ulcers. Castor oil, made from *Ricinius communis,* is a commonly used cathartic. Cayenne pepper (*Capsicum annum*) is used to aid in digestion because it is believed to stimulate gastric acid production. A tincture of cayenne pepper is applied to the skin to treat rheumatism and neuralgia. Chicory (*Cichorium intybus*), used for centuries as a coffee extender, is used as a diuretic and laxative (Touchstone, 1983).

Other Cajun folk remedies include the use of baking soda to relieve "grease gut" and as a method for "getting the fire out" of the stomach. Hog lard is used as a base for salves and is mixed with camphor for use as a chest rub. Burgoo is a corn porridge used to keep "a sick stomach from turning over." The Cajuns also frequently use gelatin made by boiling cowhides, bones, and hoofs in order to produce a hard, transparent, colloidal protein. Gelatin is given to the very ill to eat and used as a base for soups (Touchstone, 1983).

Greek Immigrant Folk Practices

Greek immigrants, many of whom settled in the north-central United States, traditionally use a folk healing practice called *matiasma*. *Matiasma* is a term used to describe the beliefs and practices surrounding the prevention, diagnosis, and treatment of the "evil eye," an illness thought to be an intentional or unintentional result of envy or admiration. Blue-eyed people are believed to be particularly capable of "casting the eye," as are older women. Children are thought to be more susceptible to the attack, and "the eye" also is thought to be able to harm inanimate objects, plants, and animals. The usual method of detecting *matiasma* is to place olive oil in a glass of water; if the oil forms a drop, the eye is believed to have been cast. Common symptoms that result from receiving "the eye" include lethargy, headache, fever, chills, and stomachache.

Special Considerations

Folk remedies for *matiasma* include wearing protective charms such as blue beads (thought to reflect the evil eye), amulets made from the wood of a saint's statue or monastery, and religious medals, garlic, or a dead individual's teeth. Behaviors used to avoid the evil eye include spitting three times after paying someone a compliment and making the sign of the cross (Tripp-Reimer, 1983).

Hmong Folk Practices

The Hmong are an Asian cultural group originating primarily in the northern hills of Laos. When North Vietnam took control of Laos, hundreds of thousands of Hmong fled to refugee camps in Thailand; from there, approximately 100,000 relocated to the United States, bringing their unique language, cultural practices, and healthcare beliefs with them (Smith, 1997a). They believe in supernatural beings that cause both good and bad fortune and also that each person has a soul, or even several souls. A person is thought to become sick when the soul attempts to leave the body. If a person becomes unconscious, the soul is believed to have left the body and will not return unless brought back by the *txi neng*, or shaman. With many Hmong converting to Christianity after their arrival in the United States, the use of shamans has decreased but still exists (Cheon-Klessig, Camilleri, Mc Elmurry, & Ohlson, 1988; Gervais, 1996; Smith, 1997a, 1997b; Westermeyer & Her, 1996).

Mysterious deaths of seemingly healthy Hmongs, known as Sudden Unexpected Nocturnal Death Syndrome (SUNDS), first were reported in 1977. Medical research has provided no adequate explanation for these sudden deaths. Adler (1995) interviewed 118 Hmong men and women and found that they believe that SUNDS is caused by nocturnal spirit encounters or attacks by evil spirits.

Special Considerations

The Hmong have a unique value and belief system, and their healthcare practices are based on a combination of tradition and belief in the supernatural. A common practice among the Hmong is the use of folk medicine (Shadick, 1993). A study of Hmong refugees in a metropolitan area revealed that almost every household practiced folk medicine, frequently using herbs or consulting with an herbalist (Cheon-Klessig et al., 1988). Several specific treatments are used, such as boiling *ntiv,* an herbal plant, with a chicken and drinking the soup several times a day following childbirth. To heal broken bones, plants are boiled with chicken blood and applied to the area for several days. Hmong shamans are perceived to have the power and capabilities to heal almost any illness or disease. If one ritual does not cure, then another is tried until a cure is found.

Homeopathic Medicine

The term *homeopathy* is derived from the Greek words *homeo* (similar) and *pathos* (suffering from disease). Homeopathy traces its roots to Hippocrates and the "law of similars." In the 4th century B.C., Hippocrates was reported to have said that, "through the like, disease is produced, and through the application of the like, it is cured" (Ullman, 1991). The concept of similars has Eastern roots, as well. The ancient martial art aikido is based on the principle that by blending and flowing with the force of the attacker, a person can throw the attacker to the ground without much effort. In a similar way, homeopathic medicines are chosen for their ability to match the symptoms of the ill person, thereby going *with* rather than *against* the body's effort to heal itself. Stewart Brand, editor of the *Whole Earth Catalog,* calls homeopathy "medical aikido" (Ullman).

The "law of similars" was rediscovered in the 1790s by the German physician Samuel Hahnemann. Through experimentation on himself, Hahnemann found that Peruvian bark, which contains quinine and was used to treat malaria, caused malaria-like symptoms if taken by people who did not have malaria. He then began to experiment with other substances from plants, animals, and minerals and found that they also could treat the same symptoms that they would cause. The information from this experimentation was carefully recorded and makes up the homeopathic *Materia Medica,* a listing of medicines and their indications for use (Collinge, 1996; Health and Human Services Dept., 1992).

Hahnemann also postulated that people possess a "vital force." He believed that the vital force was the organizing, enlivening energy that keeps people healthy. Because this vital force is affected by the energetic qualities of homeopathic remedies, homeopathy often is referred to as a form of energetic medicine. "Vital force" is a concept similar to that of *ch'i* in traditional Chinese medicine or *prana* in Ayurveda. Hahnemann believed that when this vital force is aroused to a higher level, the body can then use its own inner resources to alleviate symptoms. The remedies of homeopathy are not selected to support the body or attack pathogens. Instead, the goal is to provoke or challenge the vital force to a higher level to eliminate the symptoms and promote healing (Collinge, 1996; Health and Human Services Dept., 1992).

Constantine Hering, MD (1800–1880), considered to be the father of American homeopathy, was one of the first to observe the ways in which healing progresses. He made three observations of the healing process (referred to as "Hering's Law of Cure"), which he believed should be understood together in a unitary pattern. First, he observed that the human body seeks to externalize disease, to dislodge it from more serious, internal levels to more superficial, external levels. For example, asthmatics often develop skin rashes, which are attributed to the healing process. Hering's second observation was that healing progresses from the top of the body to the bottom. Thus, a person with arthritis in many joints generally will notice relief in the upper part of the body before the lower part. An understanding of this aspect of healing is thought to assist homeopaths in differentiating true cures from temporary relief or a placebo response. The third observation was that healing proceeds in reverse order of the appearance of symptoms. Therefore, the most recent symptoms experienced will be the first to be healed (Collinge, 1996).

An estimated 15% of all physicians in the United States practiced homeopathy in 1900 (Health and Human Services Dept., 1992). However, the practice of homeopathy declined dramatically in the United States following the publication of the Flexner Report in 1910, which established guidelines for the funding of medical schools and favored schools approved by the American Medical Association (Health and Human Services Dept.).

Homeopathic Diagnosis

In homeopathic diagnosis, the focus is on the symptoms themselves. Symptoms are viewed as the body's attempt to adapt and restore balance, or homeostasis, in the face of an infection or other stress on the body. A conventional medical diagnosis is not made; rather, a "symptom picture" is delineated based on the patient's perceptions. The symptom picture is then matched with a remedy.

Homeopathic Treatment

Three broad types of treatments or remedies exist in homeopathic medicine: acute, chronic, and constitutional. An acute remedy is one given for an acute set of symptoms in which a prompt response is needed. In acute diseases, relief is expected within a few hours to a day or two. A chronic remedy is given for more longstanding problems. The length of time for a cure is determined in part by how long the person has had the symptoms; relief may take as long as three months to two years. After a person has recovered from acute or chronic symptoms, a constitutional remedy may be given to strengthen resistance to developing symptoms in the future. The constitutional remedy works slowly and is thought to strengthen the body in a more diffuse way. It also addresses all of the patient's symptoms, vulnerabilities, and unique personality and genetic characteristics (Collinge, 1996; Ernst & Kaptchuk, 1996; Ullman, 1991).

Homeopathic treatment is a highly individualized treatment modality. Two people with the same disease typically have unique patterns of symptoms. A principle of treatment is to treat according to the patient's responses rather than according to the cause of the disease. Therefore, the cause of the disease does not need to be known in order to treat the patient (Collinge, 1996).

Proponents of homeopathy believe that modern, technologically based medicine and the overuse of pharmaceuticals carry risks of unknown long-term effects. They assert that modern medicine actually may interfere with the body's own efforts to heal by artificially suppressing the symptoms. Modern medical treatment is believed to weaken the vital force (Collinge, 1996).

Homeopathic Remedies

Homeopathic remedies are drawn from nature and include herbs, animal products, and minerals. They usually are administered in the form of pills that are dissolved under the tongue. The remedies are prepared through the process of potentization, which involves repeatedly diluting and shaking a remedy until an extremely dilute amount remains. Very dilute remedies are believed to act longer, have a deeper effect, and require fewer doses. The dilution of these substances sometimes can be further diluted to the degree that there are no remaining molecules of the original tincture in the remedy. Proponents of homeopathic medicine believe that the subtle energetic qualities of the original substance are somehow acting upon the energetic qualities of the person taking the remedy (Collinge, 1996). Contemporary homeopath George Vithoulkas (1980) explained microdose cures by defining the human body as "a magnificent cybernetic system which has the inherent capacity to respond to changes with the most efficient response" and noted that "nature uses as little as possible of anything" (p. 45). Sharma (1986) theorized that the small doses used in homeopathy are able to cross the blood-brain barrier and cellular and nuclear membranes. He also theorized that a person's vital force is sensitive to submolecular homeopathic medicines.

Various homeopathic substances have been incorporated into conventional medicine. Nitroglycerin first was used as a medicine by a homeopathic physician (Fye, 1986). Digitalis, gold salts (used in the treatment of arthritis), and colchicine (used to treat gout) are other homeopathic substances that are now widely used in conventional medicine (Ullman, 1991).

Special Considerations

Antidotes—substances with qualities that are thought to be capable of destroying the beneficial action of a remedy—in homeopathic medicine include coffee, camphor, mint, other strong tastes or scents, many prescription and recreational drugs, electric blankets, and even dental drilling. Homeopathic practitioners disagree about the effect of antidotes on homeopathic remedies. Many believe that antidotes should be avoided, at least for a short period of time, while taking homeopathic remedies. Others are convinced that if the correct remedy is selected, then antidotes should not be a concern (Collinge, 1996).

Variations of Homeopathic Practice—Classical Homeopathy

Classical homeopaths are distinguished from the nonclassical by their interest in identifying and using constitutional remedies. To make the in-depth assessment required to identify the person's unique constitution requires an intimate knowledge of the patient. The practitioner must get to know the patient well, usually in a two-hour-long consultation; in contrast, a nonclassical practitioner would give a certain remedy to everyone with a given ailment. A classical homeopath also adheres closely to Hahnemann's principle of "like cures like" (Collinge, 1996; King, 1996).

Single-Remedy Homeopathy

A variation of classical homeopathy, single-remedy homeopathy refers to the exclusive treatment of acute conditions using homeopathic medicine; chronic conditions are not treated. Single remedies are described in popular homeopathic guidebooks, such as *Everybody's Guide to Homeopathic Medicines* (Cummings & Ullman, 1997), and are available in health food stores and many pharmacies.

Nonclassical Homeopathy

In nonclassical homeopathy, the selection of remedies is not based on a detailed assessment of the person's unique constitution. Instead, remedies are given based on the ailment and whether it is acute or chronic in nature. Everyone with a given condition will receive the same remedy.

Often referred to as a shotgun approach, formula or combination homeopathy involves combining several remedies that are thought to be effective for the widest range of people. Two to eight different substances typically are mixed together, with the assumption that one or more of the components is likely to be right for the individual taking them. The combinations usually are aimed at the ailment they are intended to address (e.g., arthritis pain, teething pain, tension headache) (Collinge, 1996).

Research on Homeopathic Remedies

Medical historians believe that research on homeopathic substances marked the first use of clinical trials in medicine. Homeopaths test remedies through proving, a process in which healthy people are given a substance to see what symptoms it causes. If a common pattern to the symptoms in the group appears, then the substance is considered to be proved for that pattern of symptoms. For a substance to be logged into the homeopathic literature as effective for a particular symptom, it has to cure the symptom multiple times. In addition, it not only has to produce symptoms in healthy people but also must cure them in sick people (Collinge, 1996).

Evaluating the efficacy of homeopathic remedies is difficult because few methodologically sound clinical trials have been conducted. A major concern is that determining whether a negative finding reflects on the homeopathic remedy or on the skill level of the practitioner who selected the remedy is difficult (Collinge, 1996). Linde and Melchart (1998) published a meta-analysis of 32 trials (28 placebo-controlled, 2 comparing homeopathy and another treatment, and 2 comparing both) involving a total of 1,778 patients. The methodological quality of the trials was found to be highly variable, and when the analysis was restricted to the most sound methodological trials, no significant benefit of homeopathy was found.

In a double-blind clinical trial of homeopathic treatment versus placebo treatment conducted in Nicaragua, a statistically significant association was found between homeopathic treatment and shorter duration of childhood diarrhea (Jacobs, Jiminez, Gloyd, Gale, & Crothers, 1994). The effectiveness of homeopathic treatment of asthma was demonstrated by Reilly et al. (1994), who noted a decrease in symptoms by subjective patient reporting, a decrease in clinical symptoms, and an increase in function by practitioner assessment, improved pulmonary function tests, and decreased bronchial reactivity. In a double-blind, placebo-controlled clinical trial, the effectiveness of the homeopathic preparation called "Tinnitus" (at a homeopathic D60 potency) was evaluated by visual analog scales and a battery of audiologic measurements in 28 subjects. Neither the subjective scores nor the audiologic measures showed significant improvement in tinnitus symptoms in response to "Tinnitus" versus the placebo (Simpson, Donaldson, & Davies, 1998). The homeopathic remedy most frequently studied in placebo-controlled trials is *Arnica montana*. A meta-analysis of eight studies revealed that homeopathic *Arnica,* used in the treatment of tissue trauma, was no more effective than placebos (Ernst & Pittler, 1998).

Homeopathic Practice

Interest in homeopathic medicine has been growing, but little is known about patients who seek homeopathic care. In a study comparing patients receiving homeopathic services to patients surveyed in the 1990 National Ambulatory Care Survey, patients seen by homeopathic physicians were younger, more affluent, better educated, and more likely to present with long-term complaints (Jacobs, Chapman, & Crothers, 1998). In a survey of 10 patients seeking care for the first time from nine homeopaths, 80% reported that the impetus to seek homeopathic care was that mainstream medical care had failed to improve their symptoms. Patients sought care for a wide array of largely chronic conditions, with gastrointestinal and female reproductive problems being the most common complaints (Goldstein & Glik, 1998).

An estimated 3,000 homeopathic practitioners are working in the United States (Health and Human Services Dept., 1992). Homeopathic physicians have been found to spend twice as much time with their patients, order half as many laboratory tests, and prescribe fewer drugs than conventional medical doctors (Health and Human Services Dept.). Those who are licensed to practice homeopathy in the United States vary according to state-by-state scope of practice guidelines, and three states—Arizona, Connecticut, and Nevada—have specific licensing boards for homeopathic physicians. Homeopathic practitioners include medical doctors, dentists, naturopaths, chiropractors, veterinarians, acupuncturists, physician assistants, and nurse practitioners (Health and Human Services Dept.). Skinner (1996) described his own homeopathic nursing practice and presented case studies of how homeopathic nursing care is delivered. He noted that the most common symptoms for which he is consulted are allergies, asthma, depression, anxiety, fatigue, dermatitis, menstrual disorders, menopausal symptoms, bowel disorders, and recurring infections.

Homeopathic medicine is practiced around the world, and a renaissance in its use has been observed in Europe (Ernst & Kaptchuk, 1996). In France, 32% of the population use homeopathic remedies (Bouchager, 1990). In the United Kingdom, five homeopathic hospitals are fully integrated into the National Health Service, and some 37% of all British general medical practitioners use homeopathy (Ernst, 1996). More than 2,000 homeopathic physicians are practicing in Germany, and large numbers of non-medically trained practitioners also practice homeopathy there (Ernst). In India, homeopathy is practiced in the national health service, and more than 100 homeopathic medical colleges and more than 100,000 practicing homeopathic physicians exist (Health and Human Services Dept., 1992).

Sales of homeopathic medicines also are on the rise. In 1994, Americans spent $165 million on homeopathic remedies, and sales are rising more than 20% yearly (Ernst & Kaptchuk, 1996). Of 150 new cold remedies launched in 1994, 34 were homeopathic, compared with 17 of 92 in 1992 (Ernst & Kaptchuk). Hundreds of homeopathic remedies are available to the consumer, but most have not been proven safe or effective (Glisson, Crawford, & Street, 1999).

Cost of Homeopathic Medical Treatments

Initial interviews with classical homeopathic practitioners may range from $100 to $400, and follow-up visits typically range between $50 and $100. The number of visits required varies; more visits generally are required for chronic conditions. Homeopathic remedies typically are inexpensive, usually costing $5 to $15. Most insurance companies reimburse for homeopathic physicians' services (Collinge, 1996), while reimbursement for nonphysician providers varies (Skinner, 1996).

Latin American Rural Practices

The origins of Latin American rural health practices can be traced to the European Roman Catholic Church and ancient Indians of Mexico (Kuipers, 1995). Health practices unique to this culture have persisted for hundreds of years because the population of Latin America consists of small, rural, semi-isolated communities that have experienced little immigration and, until the last 50 years, little emigration. Individuals in these communities, consequently, have retained early healing customs and continue to practice them today (Castilla & Adams, 1996).

Latin American practices are considered to be a type of folk medicine that currently is used by many Hispanic Americans who have migrated to the United States. Many of those who use Latin American health practices trace their roots to Mexico, and most live in Texas and California (Health and Human Services Dept., 1992; Kuipers, 1995). Applewhite (1995) found that elder Mexican Americans relied on modern medicine to treat serious injuries, considered traditional folk medicine preferable for treating minor illnesses, and viewed folk healing as a viable alternative in situations in which modern health care was unsatisfactory or ineffective. In a study of Mexican Americans residing in the Texas Rio Grande Valley, 44% of 213 people surveyed indicated that they had used an alternative practitioner one or more times during the previous year and that they sought herbal medicine, spiritual healing, prayer, massage, and relaxation techniques most frequently (Keegan, 1996). The majority (66%) stated that they never report visits to alternative practitioners to their established primary health provider. Skaer, Robison, Sclar, and Harding (1996) explored predictors of utilization of folk medicine by 434 Mexican American women. They found that the most significant predictors of utilization were speaking Spanish as the language of preference, residing in the United States for one to five years, and having received medical care in Mexico within the prior five years. A study of the folk healing practices used by 76 HIV-infected Hispanics in inner-city New Jersey revealed that two-thirds engaged in folk healing (Suarez, Raffaelli, & O'Leary, 1996). The main desired outcomes of folk healing included physical relief (44%), spiritual relief (40%), and protection from evil (26%). The majority of those surveyed believed in good and evil spirits (74%), and among the believers, 48% stated that they felt the spirits played a causal role in their disease (Suarez et al.).

Latin Americans and Mexican Americans view health as a matter of chance and believe it to be controlled by forces in nature. Associated with this view is a belief in an external locus of control, or the belief that personal efforts are unlikely to influence the outcome of a situation. This belief system, known as *curanderismo,* is indigenous to the Mexican American community. Within this system, health and illness are viewed in a religious and social context rather than through the medical-scientific perspective of the dominant Western society (Kuipers, 1995).

Beliefs About Health and Illness

The concept of balance dominates much of the Mexican American belief system regarding the cause and treatment of illness. Good health is equated with being in proper balance with God, family, fellow human beings, and the church. For some Mexican Americans, health represents a state of equilibrium in which the forces of "hot" and "cold" and "wet" and "dry" are balanced. Illness is believed to occur as a result of imbalance in social or spiritual aspects of life, as a result of an imbalance of hot and cold or wet and dry, as a consequence of misfortune or bad luck, or as a punishment from God for evil thoughts or actions (Kuipers, 1995).

Treatment of Illness

Several layers of healers operate within the *curanderismo* folklore system of beliefs and practices. The first healer sought out is a key member of the family, usually a mother or grandmother, who is respected for her knowledge of folk medicine. Using healing practices that have been passed down in the family from mother to daughter, she treats the ill person until either recovery occurs or the illness becomes more complicated. Healers within the community are consulted next. The *jerbero* is a community-based folk healer who specializes in using herbs and spices for preventative and curative purposes. The more serious illnesses are treated by the *curandero* (*cuandera* if a female), or folk healer. The *curandero* is believed to have the "God-given" gift of healing and perceives life as being under the consistent influence of the divine will. People are thought to be born as sinners, with death being the ultimate consequence of their sins. The central focus of the folk healers' treatment is to relieve ill people of their sins. Diagnosis of illness by a *curandero* is made after a thorough assessment of all aspects of a person's life. Treatment, usually provided in the *curandero's* home, includes massage, diet, rest, practical advice, indigenous herbs, prayers, magic, and supernatural rituals. *Curanderos* usually are preferred over conventional medical practitioners primarily because they are thought to heal through the power of God and are viewed as being more personal, less dehumanizing, and more familiar with the patient and family. When all other levels of healers have been consulted and found to be ineffective, patients seek out *brujos*, or witches. The witches use several kinds of magic, such as green and black magic, imitative magic (which uses dolls), and certain foods and drinks as treatments (Kuipers, 1995).

Special Considerations

The following are four folk illnesses and unproven treatments that are unique to the Mexican American culture (Health and Human Services Dept., 1992; Kuipers, 1995; Risser & Mazur, 1995; Ruiz, 1985).

1. *Caida de la mollera,* or fallen fontanel, occurs in infants and is believed to be caused by a fall, rough bouncing, or forceful removal of the nipple from the baby's mouth. Common symptoms include excessive crying, diarrhea, fever, and loss of appetite. Remedies include pressing against the palate inside the mouth, praying, applying eggs to the head, and holding the child upside down.

2. *Mal ojo,* or "evil eye," occurs when a person who is thought to possess a special power admires a child of another and looks at, but does not touch, the child. This condition is characterized by headaches, fever, crying, loss of weight and sleep, and sunken eyes. Remedies include mixing eggs with water and placing the mixture under the head of the child's bed and having the person thought to be the source of the "evil eye" touch the afflicted child.

3. *Susto,* or magical fright, is believed to be caused by a frightening event and leads to the temporary loss of the spirit from the body. Symptoms include crying, insomnia, anorexia, nightmares, and fear. Remedies include rubbing the individual with herbs while praying, drinking herbal teas, and performing ritual cleansings (*barridas*), which are thought to restore the harmony of body and soul.

4. *Empacho* is the belief that something is stuck in the intestines, causing pain and blockage. Symptoms include indigestion, vomiting, and bloating. Remedies include body massage combined with drinking herbal teas.

Native American Practices

For many years, little attention was given to the medical practices and beliefs of Native Americans, which describes tribes residing in the continental United States. This group includes those residing on reservations and in rural areas as well as those who live in cities (Hanley, 1995).

Historically, Native Americans viewed medicine as an array of ideas and concepts that were firmly rooted in spiritual beliefs rather than in remedies and treatments alone. The traditional view of health was a harmony or balance among body, mind, and spirit and harmony with the physical, social, and spiritual environments. Although some practices were specific to certain tribes, many had a designated "medicine man" or "medicine woman" who was entrusted with ceremonies connected to birth and death and the perpetuation of tribal lore. This individual often served as the spokesperson for the group. The medicine man or woman served not only as the primitive doctor but also as the diviner, the rainmaker, the soothsayer, the prophet, the priest, and, in some instances, the chief. Sacred dances and lessons, usually told in the form of a story about animals, were a means of perpetuating tradition. Medicine men and women became healers as a result of experiencing a vision, dream, or "calling." Once called, the medicine man or woman received training from a medicine elder, usually as an apprentice. Training was considered to be complete when the candidate had practiced his or her skills publicly with success (Health and Human Services Dept., 1992; Tooker, 1979; Vogel, 1970).

Many Native American beliefs and practices are based on the Four Cardinal Directions, or Cords of Life (see Figure 3). The four directions are the south, west, north, and east. The clockwise circle represents the Spiral of Life, and the center circle represents the Universal Circle. Ceremonial circle gatherings are derived from the concept of the Universal Circle. The center of the circle contains the fire and is considered to represent the path to the Great One and the beginning of all living things on earth. Animals depicted in the universal circle are significant to the tribe, and stories in which animals play a central role often are told. The Cords of Life provide balance, harmony, and direction. Crystal vision is believed to come when a person is in harmony and balance with everything around him or her. The eagle feather, which represents duality, is believed to tell the story of life and represents concepts such as light and dark, man and woman, and life and death.

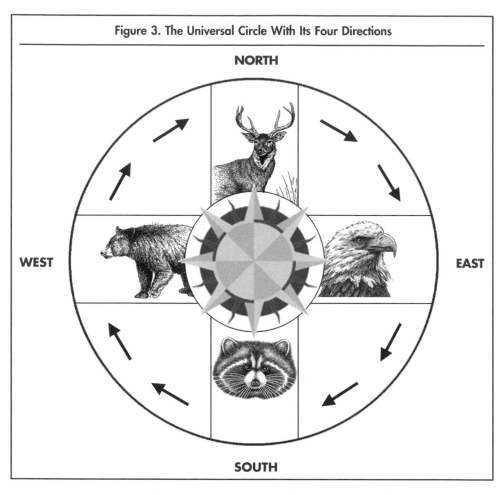

Figure 3. The Universal Circle With Its Four Directions

NORTH

WEST

EAST

SOUTH

Native Americans view the feather as the sacred symbol of the balance necessary for the Circle of Life to continue (Garrett & Garrett, 1996).

The Doctrine of Signatures has played an important role in the development of Native American medicine. "Like cures like" was the essence of this belief; thus, yellow plants were believed to relieve jaundice, and red ones were thought to influence the blood. Some parts of plants resembled the organs of the body they were designed to cure; for example, hepatica was believed to be useful in treating liver complaints, and lungwort was thought to be effective for treating pulmonary infections. Certain roots or plants were believed to be beneficial to the body because they were distasteful and injurious to the demons in the body, which were thought to cause disease. Consequently, foul-tasting medicines, emetics, and purges often were used in addition to herbal and other plant-derived remedies (Vogel, 1970).

Early settlers from Europe ignored the medical knowledge possessed by the "savages," referring to their practices as "superstitious rites." However, the early English and French colonists observed that Native Americans rarely were afflicted with ailments that they commonly contracted. In 1536, Native American women were credited with treating 100 French men who had contracted scurvy with a decoction of tree bark and sap. Through trial and error, the Native Americans found an effective remedy for scurvy, which most Europeans at that time believed to be caused by bad air. The cause was identified as a vitamin C deficiency 200 years later (Tooker, 1979; Vogel, 1970).

For the most part, the Native Americans wrote down only a very small fraction of their beliefs and practices for their own use. Instead, sacred traditions and rituals were passed from generation to generation by narrative account. The bulk of literature on Native American practices was written by anthropologists during the first decades of the 20th century (Tooker, 1979).

Native American Treatment

Although healing procedures vary from tribe to tribe, some methods are nearly universally observed. When a person becomes sick, a healer is summoned. The Native American medicine man or woman is a traditional healer with primarily naturalistic skills and typically is skilled in herbal therapy. Some medicine men or women also are shamans and are considered to be "holy." A shaman is a type of spiritual healer distinguished by the practice of journeying to nonordinary reality to make contact with the spirit world. The journey is a controlled trance state that healers induce by using repetitive sound made by drums, *chichicoya* (a gourd rattle), or movement or by consuming plant substances such as peyote or certain mushrooms (Gunn, 1995; Health and Human Services Dept., 1992).

Intuition and spiritual awareness are the healers' most essential diagnostic tools. Therapeutic methods include prayer, music, ritual purification, herbalism, massage, ceremony, and personal innovations of individual healers (Cohen, 1998).

Sweating and Purging

Common rituals prescribed by Native American healers include sweating and purging, which are intended to purify both body and spirit. In small structures, hot rocks are doused with water to create steam, which induces sweating. The sweat bath or vapor bath is thought to cleanse the body. It serves as a panacea for most diseases; herbs sometimes are taken prior to the sweat bath. Sweating continues to be practiced today, often in specially designed "sweat lodges" (Health and Human Services Dept., 1992; Vogel, 1970).

Native Americans also believe that impurities in the body should be expelled from the mouth via emetics or from the rectum via cathartics, and a large number of Native American drugs fall into these classes. One example of an emetic, ipecac, is derived from plants of the *Euphorbia* species. The Iroquois use 12 different emetics, all of which are derived from vegetables. Several act as an emetic only if taken in large doses; in moderate quantities, they serve other purposes, such as acting as a diuretic or stimulant. One such example is the "black drink" of many southeastern tribes, which consists of yaupon or cassine (Vogel, 1970).

Herbal and Other Plant-Derived Remedies

Native Americans use a host of herbal and plant-derived remedies. The roots of the cotton plant and corn smut have been used during labor either to promote contractions or to relieve pain. Both have been found to act as oxytocic agents. A decoction of wild yams is used to relieve labor pains, and the trillium species (a flower) has been called the squaw root, birth root, or papoose root because of its widespread use in childbirth. Wild sage and tea made from pennyroyal or spicebush are Native American remedies for menstrual discomfort. Although many herbal substances are used as oral contraceptives, including wild ginger, milkweed, Indian paint brush, and rosemary, their efficacy has not been scientifically verified.

Herbal remedies are used for a variety of afflictions. The bark of the white ash tree has been used as a tonic and astringent, and the tar of the balsam fir has been used for colds, coughs, and asthma. A tea of corn silk has been used as a remedy for acute bladder infections and, combined with dried bean pods, has been found to be effective in treating acute cystitis. Poultices of cornmeal have been used to treat boils, skin disorders, and infections. Corn oil is used for scaly eczema and for dandruff of the scalp. Goldenseal has been used for many purposes by Native Americans, including treatment for liver and stomach ailments, skin diseases, indolent ulcers, and gonorrhea. Witch hazel has been used for many years to relieve inflammation, soothe sore muscles, and keep legs limber (Vogel, 1970). Peppermint and spearmint have been used for soothing upset stomachs, calming nerves, and relieving headaches. Feverfew has been used as a headache remedy and an antimigraine agent. Chamomile tea has been used to soothe nervousness, and it also can be used as a skin wash to treat rashes (Garrett & Garrett, 1996).

Botanical Febrifuges

Native Americans use several botanical febrifuges, which are substances that reduce or alleviate fever. Several tribes have used dogwood bark as an antipyretic, and it contains properties similar to cinchona, a tree bark from which quinine has been extracted and used to treat malaria by South American Indians. Other Native American febrifuges include the bark of the yellow poplar and wild cherry trees and the herbs boneset and American centaury.

The Cheyennes reduced fever with a tea made from the leaves and stems of *Psoralea argophyalla*, and the Louisiana Choctaws used the root of *Verbesina virginica*, soaked in water, to make a fever extract. Wild ginger has been used to reduce typhoid fever, and an infusion of sassafras roots was used to reduce fever associated with measles (Vogel, 1970). Spicebush also has been used as a Cherokee remedy to treat measles (McWhorter, 1996).

Vermifuges

Vermifuges, or substances that facilitate the expulsion of worms and other parasites from the intestines, have been used by Native Americans for many years. The most widely used vermifuge is the pulverized root of the pinkroot, which was discovered by the Cherokee Indians. Wormseed or Jerusalem oak, which, despite its name, is an American plant, was used as a vermifuge by the Natchez. Other vermifuges include the boiled or steeped roots of wild plum, wild cherry, and horsemint (Vogel, 1970).

Massage

Massage has been an important healing procedure among many tribes. The Cherokees use massage to relieve painful menstruation, sprains, and similar conditions. The affected body part is rubbed in a circular motion, with most of the pressure being applied by the palm. Colic has been treated by rubbing the abdomen with an ointment made from the pulverized seeds of the black rattlepod. Massage using various ointments has been used to relieve pain associated with rheumatism, and in many tribes, massage is used during childbirth to relieve labor pain and aid in expulsion of the fetus (Vogel, 1970).

Special Considerations

Formal research on the efficacy of Native American healing ceremonies, herbal medicines, and Native American healers is almost nonexistent. Ailments and diseases such as heart disease, diabetes, thyroid conditions, cancer, skin disorders, and asthma reportedly have been cured by Native American doctors who are knowledgeable about the complex ceremonies (Health and Human Services Dept., 1992). Cardiovascular disease has become the leading cause of death for Native Americans and Alaska natives, and risk factors for this population include diabetes, hypertension, hypercholesterolemia, smoking, sedentary lifestyle, and obesity (Ellis & Campos-Outcalt, 1994; Muneta, Newman, Wetterall, & Stevenson, 1993). Interventions that are considered nontraditional by Native American standards, such as smoking cessation and treatment of hypertension, have been suggested to reduce mortality (Gillum, 1995). However, any treatment recommended for Native Americans must be culturally relevant and sensitive for it to be accepted (Broussard et al., 1995; LeMaster & Connell, 1994; Sanchez, Plawecki, & Plawecki, 1996).

The Indian Health Service (IHS), a federally funded program and a division of the Department of Health and Human Services, has provided medical care, educational programs, and environmental improvements that have dramatically improved Native American mortality statistics. By combining modern Western medical care with community involvement, the IHS has reduced infant mortality by 54%, maternal mortality by 65%, tuberculosis mortality by 74%, and gastrointestinal mortality by 81% since 1973 (IHS, 1997a). Fewer Native Americans now use traditional therapies; more are opting for modern Western medical treatments.

Mehl-Madrona (1999), a medical doctor, treated 16 Native American patients in conjunction with a traditional Native American healer. More than 80% had significant improvement in their symptoms and expressed satisfaction with the approach. A comparison group of Native Americans treated by a medical doctor alone had significantly lower rates of improvement and expressed a lower degree of satisfaction.

Despite wider acceptance and utilization of modern Western medical treatments among Native Americans living today, many stories still abound about seemingly impossible cures wrought by holy people. However, information on what was done is closely guarded and not readily rendered to non-Native American investigators (Health and Human Services Dept., 1992). Cook and de Mange (1995) observed several Native American tribes and found that non-Native American researchers typically experience problems gaining access to Native American cultures. Barriers to access included a lack of understanding of cultural differences, language barriers, differences in interpersonal communication, historical fear of exploitation by Native Americans, and distrust of researcher motivation (Cook & de Mange). Although research is needed to verify the efficacy of Native American treatments, the research methodology proposed must be culturally sensitive.

The majority of the 1.5 million Native Americans, members of 557 federally recognized tribes, live on or near reservations in 34 states. Most receive medical care from the IHS. With an emphasis on public health and community involvement, the IHS has been successful in providing health care to the reservation-based Native American and Alaska Native populations, who have fewer economic and educational opportunities than do other Americans. The median annual family income for Indians on reservations or tribal lands was $13,700 in 1994; among the general population, the median family income was $19,000 (IHS, 1997b). As increasing numbers of Native Americans adopt nontraditional lifestyles, diseases such as AIDS, which once were unheard of in Native American communities, are becoming more prevalent. More than one-third of all AIDS cases in Native Americans are believed to be related to IV drug usage, and 1,677 cases of AIDS have been reported to occur in Native Americans (National Native American AIDS Prevention Center, 1997).

Naturopathic Medicine

Naturopathic medicine traces its roots to ancient cultures and is considered to be the oldest medicine known to man. During the 19th century, European folk medicine was based on the philosophy of helping nature with the job of healing, and various therapies, including herbal medicines and "water cures," were used. Use of water to promote health and healing had become popular, and many spa towns flourished as a result. Large quantities of water were used, internally and externally, in conjunction with fresh air and exercise (Booth, 1994). The origins of naturopathy in the United States are attributed to Benedict Lust, who used cold water treatments and natural therapies that he learned in his native Germany and founded the first school of naturopathic medicine in New York City at the turn of the 20th century. Training at Lust's school included botanical medicine, nutritional therapy, physiotherapy, psychology, homeopathy, and manual manipulation methods. During the same period, James Foster founded a similar school in Idaho, spawning acceptance of naturopathic medicine in the Northwest (Chowka, 1997; Collinge, 1996).

Variously known as "natural therapeutics" (Baer, 1992; Chowka, 1997), the "nature cure" (Collinge, 1996), and "natural medicine" (Chowka, 1997), naturopathic medicine attracted thousands of practitioners by the 1920s, and 20 naturopathic colleges began to offer courses. However, by 1950, the practice of naturopathic medicine began to decline because of the growth of allopathic medicine, the burgeoning pharmaceutical industry, and the rise in prominence of the American Medical Association. Naturopathic medicine virtually disappeared until a resurgence of interest occurred in the 1970s (Collinge). As a growing number of Americans grew disenchanted with conventional medicine and recognized the high cost and clinical limitations of conventional treatments, many were inspired to seek "new" options and alternatives. Naturopathy and all of complementary medicine, consequently, entered a new era of rejuvenation (Baer).

Philosophy of Naturopathic Medicine

Naturopathy integrates traditional natural therapeutics, such as botanical medicine, traditional Oriental medicine (including acupuncture), hydrotherapy, and naturopathic manipulative therapy, with modern scientific medical diagnostics and standards of care. The following principles outline the unifying philosophy of naturopathy (Booth, 1994; Collinge, 1996; Health and Human Services Dept., 1992; Turner, 1990):

1. *Vis Medicatrix Naturae* (The Healing Power of Nature): The body is felt to have an inherent ability to not only heal itself and restore health but also to ward off disease. Illness is believed to be a manifestation of the organism's attempt to defend and heal itself rather than a condition caused simply by an invasion of external agents. The physician's role is to identify and remove agents that are blocking the healing process, bolster the patient's healing capacity, and support the creation of a healthy internal and external environment.

2. Treat the Whole Person: A person's health status is believed to result from a complex interaction of physical, mental, emotional, genetic, spiritual, environmental, social, and other factors. The harmonious functioning of these aspects is essential to health. Within the body, the different systems are felt to be intimately connected and dynamically balanced. "Dis-ease," or imbalance, in one part is believed to directly affect other parts of the body.

3. *Primum No Nocere* (First Do No Harm): The naturopathic physician is aware of the consequences or side effects of treatment and respects the organism's inherent ability to heal itself. It is believed that the gentler and less invasive the therapy, the less disruptive it will be to the patient.

4. *Tolle Causam* (Identify and Treat the Cause): Naturopaths believe that there is a cause for every illness and that symptoms are signals that the body is out of balance. Symptoms are an expression of the body's attempt to heal itself. Causes are believed to originate on many levels but most often are found in the patient's lifestyle, diet, habits, or emotional state. If only the symptoms are treated, the underlying causes remain, and the patient may develop a more serious condition.

5. Prevention Is the Best Cure: Naturopaths believe that health is a reflection of how people choose to live. Naturopathic physicians assist patients in recognizing their choices and in recognizing how those choices affect their health.

6. *Docere* (Doctor as Teacher): The original meaning of the word *doctor* was "teacher." A primary responsibility of the naturopathic physician is to educate and encourage self-responsibility. The physician recognizes each patient as an individual and believes that a cooperative doctor-patient relationship has inherent therapeutic value.

Naturopathic Diagnosis

Many naturopaths administer a previsit questionnaire, which serves as an aid in discussing complaints and concerns during a client's initial visit. A typical initial consultation takes approximately one hour and includes a thorough medical history and interview, which allow the practitioner to assess the patient's lifestyle, and standard diagnostic procedures, such as a physical exam. Some naturopaths use tests that are not used in conventional medicine, such as the urine indican test, which determines the degree of intestinal putrefaction (undigested and decaying food), and the Heidelberg test, which measures stomach acidity and is thought to be an indicator of digestive function (Collinge, 1996).

What happens beyond the initial consultation depends on the naturopath's specialization. A more detailed nutritional assessment may be obtained if the practitioner primarily uses a clinical nutrition approach. Likewise, in cases where the naturopath uses traditional Oriental medicine, homeopathy, or another approach, the subsequent procedures will follow in accordance with the treatment approach selected.

Naturopathic Treatment

Most naturopaths practice office-based medicine. By philosophy, they use the least invasive therapy possible and rely heavily on lifestyle assessment and counseling in order to promote healthier behaviors. Naturopaths emphasize the doctor-patient relationship and recognize that patient adherence to lifestyle recommendations is necessary for lasting improvement.

In the naturopathic perspective, healing is viewed as supporting the body's inherent mechanisms, not alleviating symptoms. For instance, the inflammatory response is considered to be one of the body's healing mechanisms and should not be routinely suppressed. Cold symptoms are allowed to flourish because the abundance of mucus is believed to flush out membranes, discharge the waste products, and promote the healing process. Naturopaths believe that the body works to follow its own innate healing strategy, and natural means are used to support these efforts. For example, naturopathic treatment of a cold may include increasing liquid intake, adding cayenne pepper to water to stimulate mucous membranes, breathing eucalyptus vapors, which act as an expectorant, and taking a homeopathic dose of onions to accelerate the body's efforts to decrease drainage (Collinge, 1996; Murray & Pizzorno, 1991).

Detoxification

Naturopaths view detoxification as one of the most important processes in promoting or optimizing overall health. Toxins are believed to play a role in the majority of chronic illnesses, and chronic illness is thought to be caused by the interaction of environmental changes, lifestyle choices, and the overuse of certain forms of medicine, such as antibiotics and anti-inflammatory agents. Many common drugs, if used indiscriminately, are believed to have a cumulative weakening effect on the body's own healing mechanisms. Most digestive disturbances are believed to be caused by food intolerance and stress. Thus, an important strategy to decrease toxic load in the body is to improve the diet, not by supplementation but by properly choosing food, and to reduce stress. Effective digestion detoxifies the body and is necessary for the expression of the body's inherent healing abilities (Collinge, 1996).

One method of detoxification is fasting, which is intended to restrict the body's intake to give the body rest and to aid in detoxification (Booth, 1994). Several regimens may be used, such as one-day fasts, during which time only water is consumed, or three- to five-day fasts, in which vegetables and juices are allowed.

Modern diets are believed to contain high amounts of toxins, which include alcohol, food additives, preservatives, and artificial sweeteners. In addition, it is thought that many people routinely consume acid-producing foods and foods to which they are unknowingly allergic, such as dairy products, wheat, corn, nuts, tomatoes, and most citrus fruits. Detoxification fasts are believed to eliminate toxic intake, remove acid-producing and allergenic foods, rest the digestive system, and stimulate the organs of elimination. Detoxification may cause looser stools, irritability resulting from unstable blood sugar levels, and foul-smelling breath, which are viewed as evidence that toxins are being effectively expelled (Weisenthal, 1997). However, fasting also has been associated with headaches, hypoglycemia, dehydration, and electrolyte imbalances (Albertson, 1996; Cerrato, 1989; Mosek & Korczyn, 1996). In a study conducted by Whitcomb and Block (1994), patients who took a 4–10 g per day dose of acetaminophen and had recently fasted were found to develop hepatotoxicity more often than nonfasting patients or those who had used alcohol.

The Vitalistic Approach

The vitalist school of thought is aligned most closely with the historic roots of naturopathy in terms of its emphasis on the body's natural healing power. At the core of the vitalistic orientation is the use of dietary change, stress reduction, and hydrotherapy. Hydrotherapy, which is one of the most commonly known naturopathic remedies, involves submersion of the body or the affected area in hot and cold water to improve circulation. Intense fluctuations in temperature are used to improve blood circulation to the stomach, liver, kidneys, and intestines and to improve digestion and elimination of metabolic waste. Hydrotherapy is believed to reduce the toxic load on vital organs and to increase immune system stimulation.

Hydrotherapy is used to treat a wide range of diseases, including ear infections and cancer (Collinge, 1996).

The Biochemical Approach

Whereas the vitalistic approach focuses on general stimulation of the body as the first line of treatment, biochemically oriented naturopaths use herbs and nutritional substances in this capacity. Substances are chosen on the basis of their biochemistry and their effects on specific disease states. In this approach, naturopathy is viewed as an alternative to conventional medicine by virtue of using substances that are considered to be more biologically correct. The biochemical approach is more predominant than the vitalistic approach, and empirical studies currently are being conducted in order to scientifically validate the biochemical naturopathic approach to treatment (Collinge, 1996).

Special Considerations

The practice of naturopathy is based on both clinical experience and scientific research. Many of the historical therapies of naturopathic medicine are being validated by modern empirical inquiry. For instance, naturopaths have used vitamin E for its antioxidant properties and protective effects against heart disease for more than 30 years, and Collinge (1996) indicated that several reports of use of naturopathic remedies (e.g., maitake mushrooms, zinc, garlic oil, acidophilus, hydrotherapy) have been published in the *Journal of Naturopathic Medicine*.

Dean Ornish, MD, director of the Preventive Medicine Research Institute at the University of California, San Francisco, has incorporated naturopathic principles into his work. He found that patients with severe coronary heart disease could not only arrest but also actually reverse their condition by following a program consisting of a low-fat diet, stress reduction strategies, and exercise (Ornish, 1990; Ornish et al., 1990).

Prospective studies have been conducted that have empirically linked specific dietary practices, such as heavy consumption of animal fat, to cancer (Giovannucci et al., 1993; Goldbohm et al., 1994). These studies lend credence to the naturopathic belief that unhealthy nutritional practices cause disease. Werbach (1993) published a compilation of thousands of abstracts of clinical studies on nutritional factors in health in a 620-page compendium. The abstracts address the influence of nutritional factors in 87 diseases. Most diseases were found to be associated with certain nutritional practices, such as high fat intake, consumption of processed foods, and a low-fiber diet.

Naturopathy also has been studied in the treatment of women's diseases. In a study of 43 women who had abnormal Pap smears, 38 returned to normal after being treated with oral nutritional and botanical supplements and with herbal suppositories (Hudson, 1993). Hudson and Standish (1993) evaluated a botanical formula as an alternative to estrogen replacement therapy. One-hundred percent of the women who received the naturopathic treatment reported a reduction in the number of menopausal symptoms, as compared to 17% in the placebo group.

In 1992, the National Institutes of Health's Office of Alternative Medicine, which was created by an act of Congress, invited leading naturopathic physicians to serve on key federal advisory panels and assist in defining research priorities. In 1994, the National Institutes of Health selected Bastyr University in Seattle, WA, as the national center for research on alternative treatments for HIV/AIDS and awarded the university $1 million of funding. Empirical studies of naturopathic approaches to treat HIV/AIDS currently are being conducted (Chowka, 1997).

Studies of utilization of naturopathic practices also have been conducted. A survey of families at a community clinic in Seattle revealed that most were choosing not to immunize their children because their naturopathic physicians advised them not to (Halper & Berger, 1981). Many viewed immunization programs as unnatural, unnecessary, and elitist.

Although naturopathic treatment is purportedly one of the safest forms of treatment (Collinge, 1996), occasional reports of adverse effects have been published. A case report described a bone marrow transplant recipient who developed hepatic zygomycosis after ingestion of a naturopathic medicine containing mucor, a mold from the genus *Rhizopus* (Oliver, Van Voorhis, Boeckh, Mattson, & Bowden, 1996). Parish, McIntire, and Heimbach (1987) published a case report of a child who sustained partial thickness burns from a garlic and petroleum jelly plaster, which had been applied at the direction of a naturopathic physician. The authors recommended that healthcare providers who are caring for children in areas where naturopathic medicine is routinely practiced be aware of the potential side effects of plasters, poultices, and other naturopathic remedies in children.

Fasting also may have adverse consequences. In a Swedish study, 6 deaths and 27 admissions to intensive care units occurred out of 123 cases in which use of alternative therapies had resulted in either a delay of diagnosis or conventional treatment or in substitution of alternative medicine for effective conventional therapy. The majority of these cases were related to fasting (Bostrom & Rossner, 1990).

Costs of Naturopathic Treatment

Naturopathic office visits are reported to cost approximately half of what conventional physician office visits cost (Collinge, 1996). The cost savings that accrue as a result of the long-term preventive focus are difficult to estimate but are believed to be quite substantial. Lower office visit costs are attributed to lower overhead because naturopaths do not require the high-technology equipment characteristic of most conventional medical practitioners. State law mandates insurance reimbursement for naturopathic treatment in Connecticut and Washington. The cost of natural substances, such as herbs, generally is much lower than pharmaceutical drugs (Chowka, 1997; Collinge).

Naturopathic Practice

Nine states officially recognize and license naturopathic physicians: Alaska, Arizona, Connecticut, Hawaii, Maine, Montana, Oregon, Utah, and Washington (Chowka, 1996). The impetus for licensing naturopathic physicians is attributed to medical consumers at the grass roots level who advocated for an affordable healthcare system that promotes wellness over disease management. To be considered for and maintain licensure, naturopathic physicians must graduate from one of the federally accredited, four-year naturopathic medical schools, pass board certification exams, and receive continuing medical education. Two of the three naturopathic medical schools in the United States, the National College of Naturopathic Medicine in Portland, OR, and Bastyr University, are fully accredited, and the third, the Southwest College of Natural Health Sciences in Scottsdale, AZ, has been accepted as a candidate for accreditation. In Utah, naturopathic physicians certified in natural childbirth are considered to be primary-care physicians with a broad scope of practice (Chowka, 1996).

A study by Cooper and Stoflet (1996) projected that the per-capita supply of naturopaths will grow by 88% between 1994 and 2010, while the conventional physician supply will grow by 16%. This predicted increase is associated with the growing number and size of naturopathic colleges as well as growth in practice opportunities and licensure. Daniels and McCabe (1994) predicted that increased utilization of natural therapies will increase the number of independent activities that the nurse performs and that the role of the nurse will shift from caregiver to healer.

Past Life Therapy

For centuries, humans have wondered what happens after death. Hindus believe that a person returns to life in a cycle of death and renewal and that a person reaps what he or she sows; a bad person in one life will come back as something unappealing, such as an insect, in the next. Orientals believe that reincarnation occurs throughout the universe, at every level of life, and is simply another way of describing the endless cycling between yin and yang (Kushi, 1992). The Tlingit of Alaska, who have a matrilinear society, believe it is important to be reborn in the family of one's mother. Conversely, the Igbo of Nigeria, who have a patrilinear society, believe that is preferable to be reborn in the family of one's father. In Nigeria, the belief in reincarnation has been widely held for many centuries but has waned somewhat in the past 30 years (Edelstein & Stevenson, 1983; Onwubalili, 1983). Some people believe that an area of the brain stores all or part of the lives they have lived and that they are able to return to past lives. The process of hypnotically returning to these past lives is called past life therapy or past life regression (Moody, 1990).

Simple Age Regression

Past life regression is believed to have evolved from the procedure called simple age regression, which is conducted in one of two ways. Simple age regression refers to the use of hypnosis to go back in time through a person's present life. Past life regression refers to going back in time to a prior life. The first type of simple age regression, called revivification, refers to the process by which the hypnotized subject relives or re-experiences the events of his or her life at an earlier age. Subjects speak and write as they did at that age. The second type of age regression, called pseudo-revivification, is characterized by the subject being able to relive scenes from an earlier age and recall memories following that age. In other words, subjects are aware that they are still in the present but are experiencing scenes from the past. Their speech, handwriting, and other characteristics do not change from those they currently possess. One characteristic of both types of simple age regression is called hypermnesia, or heightened recall, in which subconscious memory banks are being tapped during deep hypnosis and vivid recall occurs.

Simple age regression is a technique that many hypnotherapists use. A person's present phobias, conflicts, and psychological distress are thought to be rooted in the past, and prior events, especially those that occurred during childhood and have been repressed, may represent keys to understanding the present. In investigating crimes, many instances of simple age regression in which details have been described, such as recalling a license plate number in a murder case, have been documented (Goldberg, 1982).

Past Life Regression

While many hypnotherapists use simple age regression, some use the technique to take the client back to the birth experience and then suggest the next logical step, which is going back to a past life. Past life therapy is founded upon the assumption that actions and problems in previous lives determine the problems, neuroses, and phobias of a person's present life (Marriott, 1984). Most of the literature on past life experiences has been written in anecdotal fashion, and case reports or transcripts from regression sessions often are used to illustrate the process (Jue, 1996; Ramster, 1994).

The earliest accounts of individuals recalling past lives were unexpected. Moody (1990) noted that while working as a psychotherapist, he was surprised to hear hypnotized patients describe puzzling episodes during which they seemed to be transported back in time and space where they experienced a sense of identity with an individual who lived in an earlier historical period. Sometimes, the patients spoke another language or used words and phrases that clearly were different from their usual language patterns.

While accounts of past lives historically have been dismissed as bogus, Ian Stevenson, MD, a respected psychiatrist, conducted regression hypnosis on hundreds of people and concluded that a very small fraction provided verifiable accounts, which he published in the book *Twenty Cases Suggestive of Reincarnation* (1966). Audiotapes and transcripts of his interviews were given to various authorities, including anthropologists, historians, and language experts. In the 20 cases described, fraud was dismissed after careful expert analysis. The 20 people demonstrated unusual qualities during regression hypnosis, such as speaking in brogue or possessing a thorough knowledge of obscure subjects, such as trade wind patterns or the religious beliefs of the Quakers. Several regressed children were able to compute advanced mathematics or accurately describe unfamiliar processes, such as giving birth (Moody, 1990).

In recent years, past life experiences have received media attention and sparked public interest. "New Age" therapies, which became popular in the 1980s, incorporated past life regression. The Association for Past-Life Research and Therapy, which was established by 52 therapists and now has several hundred members worldwide, offers workshops and conferences and publishes the *Journal of Regression Therapy* (Moody, 1990).

The current fascination with past lives has led to an increase in the number of people seeking past life explorations. Perhaps the most common reason why people seek past life explorations is out of simple curiosity. Other reasons include self-exploration, conflict resolution, and to find answers to questions. People who seek past life explorations tend to fall into two distinct groups: the "doubting Thomases," who are intent on disproving the approach, and those with great expectations, who are utterly convinced that they have lived past lives (Goldberg, 1982).

Regression Hypnosis

Regression hypnosis usually is a lengthy process that involves substantial questioning by the therapist while the subject is deeply hypnotized. Hypnosis refers to a psychically induced sleep-like state. Hypnosis is recognized as a reputable clinical aid; since 1958, the American Medical Association has formally acknowledged the efficacy of hypnosis (Goldberg, 1982). During hypnosis, the regression therapist asks a series of questions. For instance, when the subject makes a reference to his or her surroundings, the therapist must probe for details and descriptions, using such questions as, "How are the people around you acting?" or "How are the people dressed?"

Regression hypnosis usually is performed on an individual basis; however, some accounts of group regression have been published (Moody, 1990). Individual regression is believed to produce the best results because people tend to hypnotize more deeply when they are alone. Another regression technique is called *scrying*, which is better known as crystal-ball gazing. Scrying is popular among Tibetan wise men; in this technique, the subject literally gazes into a crystal ball or some other clear depth while being hypnotically induced (Moody).

While all past life regressions are unique, several common characteristics of regression experiences have been identified (Moody, 1990; Spanos, Burgess, & Burgess, 1994):

1. Past life experiences usually are visual and consist of sensory images.
2. The scenes and events visualized seem to unfold of their own accord. Subjects feel as if they are witnessing events rather than making them up, as a day-dreamer would.
3. The imagery has an uncanny feeling of familiarity. The feelings are described as being similar to the experience of déjà vu, the feeling that one has already done or seen whatever he or she is currently experiencing.
4. A person identifies himself or herself as one of the individuals in the unfolding drama.
5. Past life emotions may be re-experienced during a regression. Emotional "re-living" may cause acute distress in the subject.
6. The experience often mirrors present issues in the subject's life. Events and situations that unfold during regression often reflect the dilemmas and conflicts faced by the subject in his or her present life.
7. Regression may be followed by an improvement in mental state. Catharsis, in which pent-up feelings finally are allowed to be expressed, often occurs during regression and will result in the subject reporting an improvement in mood following the regression session.
8. Regressions may affect medical conditions. In some instances, subjects have reported dramatic improvement or decline in physical symptoms.
9. Regressions develop according to meanings, not a historical time line. If a subject was regressed to a dozen distinct "past lives," the series of lives will occur around an emotional or relationship theme, not in the chronological sequence in which they would have been lived.

10. Past life regressions become easier with repetition.
11. Most past lives are mundane. Very rarely do subjects identify with a known historical figure; instead, the vast majority appear to live lives that were typical of the period to which they regress. Subjects claiming to have lived as well-known historical figures (especially multiple well-known figures) are likely to be fabricating their accounts.

Illness: A Reincarnationist's View

Regression therapists who believe in reincarnation have a metaphysical perspective on illness. They believe that illnesses are subconsciously chosen as a lesson and represent an altered state of awareness. Illness, therefore, shapes a person's perception of reality. For example, even a simple sore throat will change the way a person views the world. People experiencing illness, particularly catastrophic diseases such as cancer, are reassured that they will survive bodily death and are told that they will learn much about themselves on a spiritual level because of their illness experience (Moody, 1990).

Special Considerations

As noted previously, past life regression is an extension of simple age regression therapy. Practitioners believe that a fairly large number of people are able to recall prior forgotten or repressed memories from their current life under hypnosis. Often, these memories are based on actual experiences or composites of personal experiences; they also may be based on other sources, such as books that were read, movies that were seen, or stories that were heard. Regression to a past life is more complex and controversial. The Roman Catholic Church denounces the concept of reincarnation, and many people simply do not believe in the concept. Hypnotherapists performing past life regression therapy admit that some people's accounts of "past lives" may simply represent recall of earlier forgotten memories; for instance, specific details can be attributed to a forgotten family story or material learned in high school geography courses rather than a past life. Hypnotherapists also acknowledge that some people undergoing regression therapy "create" their past lives, perhaps to impress their therapist or others. However, there remain a very small number of individuals for which no such explanation exists and for whom evidence suggestive of reincarnation has been documented (Moody, 1990).

Moody (1990) noted that past life regressions are akin to exploring a mystery. Regressions may serve as a valuable tool in understanding oneself but also may leave many questions. Vivid experiences are believed by many to be "proof" of a life before life; however, like all powerful techniques of self-discovery, there are many concerns about regression therapy. The first concern is the regression therapist's qualifications. The enormous public demand for past life regression, coupled with the fact that hypnosis is a very easy procedure to learn, has created a situation in which uninformed and untrained individuals have set themselves up as "experts" in regression therapy. The limited number of licensed psychiatrists and psychologists who offer regression therapy further compounds this problem. To be properly administered, a process that psychotherapists call "working through" should follow regression therapy. In other words, once powerful emotions or memories have been liberated by regression hypnosis, a professional is needed to guide the subject in talking about those feelings and to help the person integrate them into the larger fabric of his or her life. People interested in pursuing past life explorations should ask for the hypnotherapist's credentials, verify those credentials with local licensing boards, and be wary of "therapists" who purport to *tell* a person about their past lives. Regression therapy is considered to be a method of self-exploration.

A second concern about regression therapy is the potential that certain individuals will develop an obsession with past life matters. Some people become so engrossed in their past lives that regression becomes an end in itself rather than one tool among many in the road to self-understanding. Again, only qualified regression therapists should be consulted for this therapy. Professional therapists possess the ability to diagnose and treat diverse psychiatric disorders and can identify underlying obsessive disorders.

A third concern about regression therapy is that many people seeking regression have unrealistic expectations. They believe that if only they were hypnotized and taken back to a past life, they would experience dramatic relief from annoying conflicts and problems. A related concern is the use of regression therapy as a means of escapism. The overwhelming complexity of modern life has caused many individuals to feel alienated, and regression therapy provides escapist immersion in other lives and simpler times.

People seeking regression therapy should be carefully screened for depression and low self-esteem. Depressed people and those with a low sense of self-worth tend to become infatuated with past life regression as an attempt to cure their lack of positive feelings for themselves. They can develop the attitude of, "So what if I haven't amounted to much in this life? In a past life, I was powerful, wise, and wealthy."

Regression therapy is best provided by qualified, experienced hypnotherapists. A person should only use the term *hypnotherapist* if he or she has a doctorate as a health professional, such as a psychologist or psychiatrist. These professionals can properly screen individuals for regression therapy, administer hypnotic regression, and provide psychological support. The term *hypnotist* refers to those without professional training other than hypnosis training, which typically is obtained by participating in a week-long program.

Regression therapy is a form of therapy that does not lend itself well to traditional empirical research approaches. Instead, case studies and studies of attitudes of people who believe in reincarnation have been reported in the literature. Exley, Sim, Reid, Jackson, and West (1996) studied attitudes toward organ donation and found that members of the Sikh community rejected donation because of their belief in reincarnation. A case report of the use of past life therapy was published by Goldberg (1982), who reported successfully treating dental phobia using regression therapy.

Stevenson (1983) examined 79 American children who purported to remember previous lives. Few were found to make verifiable statements, and those who did often spoke of deceased members of their own families. Most past life accounts were thought to be derived from fantasies.

Shamanism

In ancient times, many cultures believed that people could communicate with the heavens and travel physically to the spirit world. The Koryaks of Asia thought that the heavens could be reached by climbing through an opening in the sky or by following the path of an arrow shot upward. The word *shaman* comes from the Tungas tribes of Siberia and refers to a man or woman who possesses a specific type of spiritual power (Cowan, 1993). Shamans voluntarily enter an altered state of consciousness and travel to other realms to serve their communities (Walsh, 1989). Shamanism is practiced all over the world, and anthropologists believe that shamanic traditions were carried to other parts of the globe by migratory peoples. Historically, shamans worked in a trance state and were considered to be visionary healers. In recent years, however, the word *shaman* has been applied loosely—and often inaccurately—to many types of spiritual and healing practices associated with tribal cultures (Cowan; Stein, 1991).

Shamanism is a way of viewing reality and a method or technique for functioning within that view of reality. The shaman perceives the universe differently than other people and has personal experiences in the universe that seem to transcend those of other people. The core elements of shamanism found in most cultures with a documented shamanic tradition are (a) shamans can voluntarily enter a unique visionary state of consciousness, (b) during this state, they experience a journey into nonordinary realms of existence, and (c) the journey enables shamans to acquire knowledge and power for their own use and for others in their communities (Cowan, 1993; Harner, 1990). These three features comprise what many shamanic practitioners today call *core shamanism*. Because the nonordinary realms are immaterial and largely imaginal, shamans speak of them as spirit realms, and the entities encountered there are considered spirits. In healing, for instance, a shaman may journey into nonordinary reality to treat the invisible, spiritual nature of the illness (Cowan).

Shamanism is a worldwide phenomenon that has survived in various forms beyond the hunting-fishing-gathering societies of 20,000 years ago. Campbell (1983) stated that shamanism is "the essential component of an immemorial tradition, to which a number of characteristics are attached, of which some may be accented in one region, others in another, but always in relation to the vocation that calls a man or woman to become a walker between the worlds of ordinary and nonordinary reality" (p. 157).

Shamans

Men or women are designated as shamans when they have demonstrated the ability to journey into nonordinary reality, receive help from spirit guides, and return with some knowledge or power to serve others in the community. Authentic shamans are believed to be "called" to the profession, and a person usually becomes aware of his or her shamanic abilities following a traumatic initiatory crisis, such as a near-death experience or out-of-body experience. Shamans are believed to have the ability to make repeated journeys into the "Otherworld" at will, the ability to make contact with spirit guides in that world, and the ability to "work magic" or control reality in ways that are considered extraordinary by community standards (Cowan, 1993).

The most common method of entering the shamanic state of consciousness is to listen to a mesmerizing sound, such as the monotonous beating of a drum, the clicking of sticks, or the shaking of a rattle, or to engage in a repetitious activity, such as clapping, chanting, or dancing (Walsh, 1996). What distinguishes a shaman from other mystics is the journey into the "Otherworld" and trust in the spirits for acquiring the power and wisdom that the shaman will share with the community in the form of shamanic services when he or she returns. Shamanic services are many and varied and include divination, healing, dream interpretations, rites of passage, soul retrieval, and other personal or communal rituals a client may request (Kalweit, 1988).

Shamanic View of Healing and Dying

Shamans use a process called divination to diagnose illness. Divination is performed in different ways but refers to discovering hidden information by supernatural methods. Siberia's Samoyed shamans throw a stick in the air and observe the position of the stick when it lands, which they believe indicates the nature of the illness. Shamans in Melanesia gaze into quartz crystal and then make a diagnosis. Eskimo shamans use a pendulum while asking questions; if the pendulum swings in one direction, the answer is "yes," whereas swinging in the other direction means "no" (Stein, 1991).

In shamanic belief, the cause of illness is found at the spirit level and is attributed to a loss of soul or power or to the intrusion of an enemy spirit. The shaman communicates with the spirit world to diagnose and treat a problem. If a soul is lost, the shaman will travel to the "Otherworld" to retrieve it. If an intruder is believed to be present, the shaman will remove it, usually by sucking it out. The sucking or extraction is accomplished by sucking the affected body part, either via a tube or directly with the mouth. The shamans are careful, however, to not draw what they believe to be the harmful spirit into their own stomachs (Cowan, 1993; Stein, 1991).

In many cultures, the shaman also uses a sacred medicine bundle. The bundle contains objects used for healing, such as crystals, pebbles, dried plants, bones, and feathers. Sacred drugs are used throughout the world, and the shamans sometimes use these drugs to gain access to the spirit world. In South America, shamans drink *caapi*, which is brewed from the banisteriopsis vine. Users purport that transport to the "Otherworld" occurs rapidly and that they can even journey to the beginning of time. Séances, or public ceremonies, are conducted by shamans and are considered to be important for healing. Both the shaman and audience take part through drumming, singing, and dancing, and sacred drugs sometimes are consumed, as well (Stein, 1991). In South American Indian cultures, ritual tobacco use, which is aimed at achieving acute nicotine intoxication, is used to enhance shamanic practice (Wilbert, 1991).

In ancient cultures, the belief that people lived another life when their soul passed on to another body prevailed. Deaths at an early age were common, but death was not feared because the souls of men were believed to be immortal. Books of the Dead, written in many early societies, described the stages and experiences that were believed to encompass the transition from earthly consciousness to the "Otherworld" and then back again into another body. The Celtic people viewed shamans as primary explorers and mapmakers for this process. The shamans shared their knowledge of the "Otherworld' with other members of their communities, and psychologically, this knowledge reassured the living that the territory of death had been explored and even charted (Cowan, 1993).

Special Considerations

Dobkin de Rios and Winkelman (1989) suggested that Western cultural avoidance of shamanism has inhibited understanding of shamanic phenomenon and that research is needed to further explore altered states of consciousness. Anecdotal accounts of shamanic practice have been published, including the account of a psychotherapist who used shamanism herself to transcend the pain of childbirth and, in another example, to break through to a deeper understanding of a difficult patient (Damery, 1997). Aspects of shamanic healing, including what Baker (1992) called "creative visualization," have been used during pregnancy and childbirth to increase awareness of the psycho-spiritual aspects of giving birth.

Western influences, the rise of Buddhist monasticism, and the growth of organized religion led to the repression and denouncement of shamanic practice (Ortner, 1995). The Catholic church considered shamanism "witchcraft," and, as a result, many shamans were killed in the 1500s during the Spanish Inquisition. Traditional shamanism continued to be practiced in certain areas, mostly among the Laplanders and others in the northernmost part of Europe, until the 1930s when Christian missionaries arrived. Shamanism still is commonly practiced in some remote parts of Siberia and Australia. In Australia, the shaman is known as *karakdi* or "clever man" (Stein, 1991).

Today, people in modern societies are developing a renewed interest in shamanic techniques. Redfield (1993) published a bestseller titled *The Celestine Prophecy,* which contained shamanic philosophies and stimulated a growing interest in spiritual awareness. Rioux (1996) advocated using shamanic healing techniques in addiction counseling. He postulated that recovery from addiction represents a transformation of consciousness, which he describes as "participatory holism." Winkelman (1990) called modern-day shamans "magico-religious practitioners" and noted that their practice is characterized by inducing altered states of consciousness and power relationships. Huichol Indian shamans have kept their shamanic traditions alive and continue to perform Huichol ceremonies, vision quests, and pilgrimages to "places of power" (Foundation for Shamanic Studies, 1997).

Many people seek shamanic practice because of dissatisfaction with conventional medicine, and claims have been made that shamanic healing was effective when traditional therapies were not. Stein (1991) offered one explanation for this phenomenon: shamans' "position of authority with the spirits allows them to make strong suggestions for healing. Their presence shifts the patient's attention from the illness to the likelihood of getting better" (p. 99). Medical researcher Jeanne Achterberg (1985) suggested that, because shamans do not do anything that directly changes body chemistry, they teach patients to use imagery to become well. She compared shamans' work with guided imagery and the placebo effect, in which a healing response is triggered by a belief or expectation that a treatment will work. The Foundation for Shamanic Studies (1997) reported that "open-minded Westerners are beginning to discover that shamanic methods can yield astonishing results in problem-solving and healing, for themselves and for others" (p. 1).

There is much concern, however, that many currently practicing "shamans" use fraud and sleight of hand to produce "miracles" and that many do so at the emotional and financial expense of the patient. The vulnerability of patients with catastrophic illnesses, such as cancer and AIDS, makes them a prime target for self-serving "shamanic" practitioners. Unfortunately, no licensing or regulatory body oversees shamanic practice in the United States. Patients who are interested in receiving shamanic healing should be informed about the history and practice of shamanism and be cautioned about possible exploitation.

Tibetan Medicine

Tibetan medicine has been practiced for thousands of years and is based on the medical teachings of the Buddha. The teachings were complied into four texts, called the Four Tantras. The first is known as the Root Tantra, which is a short text that outlines the whole medical teaching. The second is the Explanatory Tantra, which deals with formation of the human body, its functions, and the characteristics of disorders. The Oral Tradition Tantra describes the causes and symptoms of disease and outlines methods of treatment. The fourth text, the Last Tantra, contains instructions on diagnostic methods and the manufacture of medications. The Four Tantras are studied with the help of visual aids in the form of trees, which consist of three roots, nine trunks, and 42 branches. Each trunk is divided in two to represent a healthy body in a balanced state and an unhealthy body in an imbalanced state. A healthy body also is thought to contain seven physical constituents: nutritional essence, blood, flesh, fat, bone, marrow, and regenerative fluid. A person is considered to be healthy when balance exists in the three humors: *rLung,* which is symbolized by the bird and known as wind, motility (*qi*), or movement; *mKhris-pa,* which is symbolized by the snake and known as bile or heat; and *Bad-kan,* which is symbolized by the pig and known as phlegm or moisture (Donden, 1986).

Illness: The Tibetan View

In the Tibetan system, there are believed to be more than 84,000 different types of afflictive emotions, such as desire and hatred, that have corresponding effects on human beings; thus, 84,000 different types of disorders can occur. These disorders have been further condensed into 404 recognized illness states (Donden, 1986).

Disorders are classified by location in the body, type, and environmental factors and include the following (Donden, 1986):

- 101 disorders that are under the strong influence of actions (*karma*) in previous lifetimes

- 101 disorders of this lifetime, which have their causes in an early period of the life and manifest later
- 101 disorders involving spirits
- 101 superficial disorders, which result from dietary imbalances or behavior patterns.

When the three humors are in balance, health is maintained and disease remains in a dormant state. When an imbalance among the humors occurs, they become entities of disease and harm the body. Illness is believed to arise from two different causes—proximate and distant. The proximate causes are wind, bile, and phlegm. When a disorder of bile occurs, the seven physical constituents are heated. When a phlegm disorder occurs, it reduces or smothers body heat. Wind is common to both cold and heat and assists whichever is more prominent. Many distant causes of illness exist and frequently relate to the environment (Donden, 1986; Finckh, 1981).

Diagnosing Illness

In Tibetan medicine, a diagnosis is made by touch, by feeling the pulses. The Tibetan doctor, who also is a lama (an extraordinary person with spiritual power), places his hands on the patient's radial artery and uses specific fingertip locations to "read" a specific major organ in the body (see Figure 4). The material basis of the body, known as the five elements of wood, fire, earth, iron, and water, produces certain types of pulse beats during specific seasons. The Tibetan doctor

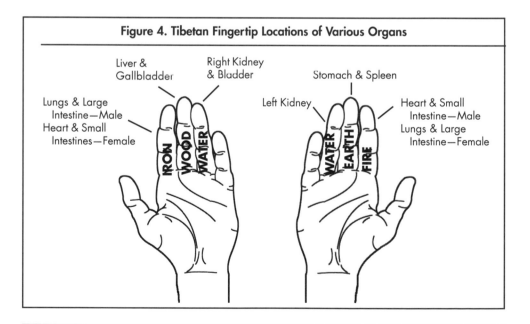

Figure 4. Tibetan Fingertip Locations of Various Organs

palpates these locations on the fingers, evaluates the quantity and quality of the pulses, and makes a diagnosis (Donden, 1986; Finckh, 1981; Steiner, 1989).

Questioning is another diagnostic technique that is used in Tibetan medicine. Patients are asked questions about the conditions that give rise to specific diseases; for instance, if a patient has symptoms of a wind disease, the doctor will ask questions about mobility. A third diagnostic technique is urinalysis. The urine is examined three times—when it is hot, lukewarm, and completely cool—and the doctor notes the urine's color. A bile disorder will manifest as an orange color, a red color indicates a blood disorder, and a rust color indicates a lymph disorder. If the urine is brown, it indicates a complex disorder of the three humors—wind, bile, and phlegm. A foul urine odor is thought to indicate a heat disorder, and if no odor is present, then a cold disorder exists. Froth or bubbles are believed to indicate a wind disorder. In addition to being used as a diagnostic technique, urinalysis is used to estimate prognosis (Donden, 1986; Rapgay, 1986).

Tibetan Medical Treatment

Tibetan medicine consists of internal medicine, which incorporates diet and behavioral interventions, and external medicine, which includes various bodywork therapies (Donden, 1986). The Tibetan medical approach encompasses spiritual, psychological, and physical aspects when diagnosing ailments (Tokar, 1999). Behavior and diet modifications are hallmarks of Tibetan treatment, and specific dietary recommendations are made based on seasonal considerations. For instance, when the weather is cold, phlegm is believed to accumulate in the body; therefore, the three tastes of hot, bitter, and astringent should be eaten to reduce the phlegm accumulation. Phlegm also is reduced by exercising (walking and running) and washing with lentil powder instead of soap (Donden).

Tibetan meditation, called *samatha*, is used to promote a state of calm. Meditation is performed at sunrise, with the individual facing west, and sunset, with the individual facing east. The calm state achieved by meditation is believed to move the wind humor through the body, which, in turn, moves the blood through the body (Hollifield, 1998).

Fomentation, or the application of compresses to affected body parts, is a commonly practiced external medicine treatment that is believed to remove phlegm from the body. The compresses usually are hot and may contain various plant substances. Also included among external treatments are hydrotherapy and massage, both of which promote movement and motility. Hydrotherapy is used to remove bile, and massage is thought to alleviate wind diseases. Symptoms of wind diseases include restlessness, insomnia, dizziness, unbalanced emotions, depression, stiffness, and head and back aches. Massage may incorporate oils or an ointment rub, or *kunyi*, which is an herbal paste or liniment used to rub acupuncture points on the body. Other types of Tibetan massage include stroking in long, longitudinal strokes (also called effleurage); rubbing in a vigorous circular motion, creating friction; kneading; and acupressure, which involves deep, circular, manual pressure massage (Hollifield, 1998).

Acupuncture can be used with or without moxibustion, a procedure in which the herb moxa is burned at an acupuncture point. In traditional Tibetan medicine, the moxa from the *Artemesia argii* or *Vulgaris sensis* plants is collected and prepared by the lama. Tibetans believe that the *qi* (energy) of the lama affects the quality of the moxa that is gathered. Tibetans use moxibustion treatments for heat deficiencies, digestive problems, water accumulation, and various other disorders. The locations of the acupoints are patterned in a system similar to the meridian system used in traditional Chinese acupuncture. However, in the Tibetan system, the moxa points are not associated with points on meridians but rather are simply points on the body at which moxa treatments are given. Moxa is applied via four techniques: *tso wa*, a cancer treatment that involves burning large cones of moxa on the skin and removing them before the skin is burned; *sek pa*, a treatment for phlegm disorders in which the moxa is allowed to burn down to the skin to the point that blisters result; *so wa*, an indirect treatment for various disorders of *qi* and blood in which moxa is rolled in mulberry bark paper and placed on the skin to heat it; and *dik pa*, a treatment used for children and the very ill in which a slow transfer of heat is delivered via wrapped moxa held above the skin (Hollifield, 1998).

Special Considerations

Very little empirical research has been published on the efficacy of traditional Tibetan medical practices. Ryan (1997) conducted a randomized, controlled study in a community in Northern India where Tibetans are exposed to both traditional Tibetan and Western medicine. He compared the Tibetan practice of massage and compress application for arthritis treatment to the Western medical practice of prescribing anti-inflammatory agents and found the indigenous Tibetan treatment to be significantly more effective than the Western treatment for improving limb mobility and comfort.

Traditional Tibetan medicine continues to be practiced today, mostly in Tibet and northern India and by those who originated in those areas and migrated to others, such as the Buddhist monks (Begley, 1994). Some patients who have become dissatisfied with Western medicine have turned to Tibetan practitioners for medical care, and many of those patients have begun adopting Buddhist religious practices as well.

Traditional Oriental Medicine

The term "Oriental medicine" often is used interchangeably with "Chinese medicine." Bao (1992) noted that the nomenclature is unclear and can result in improper usage of terms. Traditional medicine of China should be called "traditional Chinese medicine" rather than the frequently used "Chinese medicine" because the term "Chinese medicine" fails to distinguish between traditional and modern Chinese medicine. Traditional Oriental medicine is rooted in Chinese culture and encompasses many variations, including Japanese, Korean, Cambodian, and Vietnamese.

The origins of classical Oriental medicine are obscure, buried in thousands of years of tradition. The third ruler of China, Huang Ti, is believed to have authored the first and most important textbook on the subject, titled *The Yellow Emperor's Classic of Internal Medicine (Huang Ti Nei Ching Su Wen,* herein referred to as the *Nei Ching),* around 2597 B.C. Chinese medicine is derived from Chinese religion. At their core, both have the same ingredients: the Tao, yin and yang, the universal energy ch'i, and the five elements of wood, fire, earth, metal, and water (Reisser, Reisser, & Weldon, 1987).

The Tao

The Tao, or "the way," stresses the importance of process and change, which is illustrated by nature's continuous cycles. Day becomes night, winter turns to spring, wet becomes dry, and so on, all in observable patterns. In Taoism, human beings, who are seen as totally dependent on nature, are urged to live in harmony with these cycles and thus be "one" with the Tao. The individual who does so is promised success and long life, while the person who challenges nature's cycles will experience disease and an early death (Reisser et al., 1987).

Yin and Yang

Yin and yang are believed to be the two fundamental forces that generate all of the transformations in the universe. These forces are bipolar; yin and yang literally mean "shady" and "sunny" sides of a hill (Fulder, 1987). Yin and yang have evolved to encompass a wealth of characteristics (see Figure 5). All events in nature and in human beings are believed to be influenced by the ever-changing interplay of these forces. Neither is believed to exist in an absolute state, and small amounts of each are contained in the other, as illustrated by the ancient symbol T'ai-chi T'u, the "Diagram of the Supreme Ultimate" (see Figure 6).

The *Nei Ching* applies the interaction of yin and yang to the human body. The inside of the body is yin; the surface, yang; the front, yin; and the back, yang.

Figure 5. Characteristics of Yin and Yang	
Yin	**Yang**
Dark	Light
Moon	Sun
Night	Day
Feminine (wife)	Masculine (husband)
Below	Above
West/north	East/south
Metal	Wood
White/black	Green/red
Rest	Movement
Spring/summer	Autumn/winter
Interior	Exterior
Contraction	Expansion

Figure 6. The Ancient Chinese Symbol T'ai-chi T'u

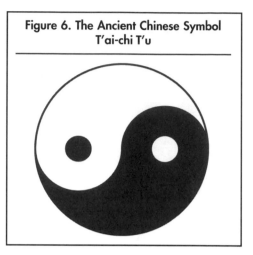

Each major organ of the body is designated as yin or yang, depending on which force dominates its function. Health is defined as the state in which yin and yang are in perfect, dynamic balance over a period of time. Disease or illness occurs when an excess of yin or yang accumulates in specific body organs (Fulder, 1987).

Ch'i

Ch'i refers to a universal, invisible life force energy that is believed to flow through all living organisms. Ch'i reputedly is inhaled with air and extracted from food and drink. Once inside the body, it finds its way to a network of 12 invisible channels, called meridians, each of which is associated with a particular organ and shares that organ's yin or yang polarity. The 12 meridians are duplicated symmetrically on each side of the body and divided into closely associated pairs (Fulder, 1987).

Disease or illness occurs when the flow of ch'i is obstructed or excessive in any area, which disrupts the balance of yin and yang. Healing occurs when balance is restored. In the *Nei Ching,* specific diseases, such as pneumonia or diabetes, do not exist. Instead, imbalances of yin and yang are referred to by names such as "injuries to the stomach."

Diagnosing Illness

In diagnosing the cause of an illness or disease, the individual's complaints, appearance, and breathing patterns are evaluated, and the pulses are examined. At each wrist, the radial pulse is divided into three zones, each of which has a superficial and deep position. Twelve pulse locations correspond to the 12 meridians and are believed to communicate information about organ imbalances to the examiner (see Figure 7). Each pulse position is carefully felt and characterized as full, weak, floating, slippery, or wiry. Pulses are interpreted in the context of several factors, including the time of day, season of the year, and gender of the individual. This diagnostic process may take 30 minutes or more (Reisser et al., 1987; Wallnöfer & von Rottauscher, 1985).

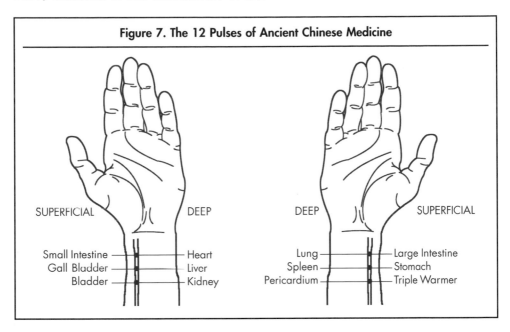

Figure 7. The 12 Pulses of Ancient Chinese Medicine

SUPERFICIAL   DEEP   DEEP   SUPERFICIAL

Small Intestine — Heart   Lung — Large Intestine
Gall Bladder — Liver   Spleen — Stomach
Bladder — Kidney   Pericardium — Triple Warmer

Traditional Oriental Medicine Treatment

Once a diagnosis is made, the *Nei Ching* offers five basic approaches to therapy. The first is treatment of the spirit, which guides the individual toward the Tao in the practice of a modest, tranquil way of life through meditation and healing exercise. The second and third are dietary and herbal therapies, the fourth is acupuncture, and the fifth is massage.

Internal and External Exercise

The use of physical exercise and meditation as therapeutic techniques can be traced to about 1000 B.C. in China (Health and Human Services Dept., 1992). Qigong refers to the art and science of using breath, movement, and meditation to cleanse, strengthen, and circulate the vital life energy and blood. Ancient Taoists called meditation "internal exercises," which were created after careful study and application of the physical laws of nature and the natural principles of healing. Physical exercise and meditation methods were designed to coax the diseased body parts back to their natural order (i.e., to health). When practiced daily, meditation and physical exercise are believed to promote freedom from disease and pain and create a sense of well-being (Reid, 1994).

Meditation

Meditation restores access to what the Taoists call the "original mind" and promotes a relaxed state of mind that not only calms and rejuvenates but also focuses attention to other nonrational, nonsensory sources of information and knowledge. During meditation, mental static, or internal dialogue, which is generated by the rational, linear thinking of the cerebral cortex, is stilled and silenced (Reid, 1994).

The two primary methods used in meditation are *jing* (quiet, stillness, calm) and *ding* (concentration, focus). The methods used in meditation focus on three levels: essence (body), energy (breathing), and spirit (mind). Although various specific techniques can be used, the following techniques are characteristic of Taoist meditation, which frequently is used in traditional Oriental medicine (Reid, 1994).

1. Adopt a comfortable, balanced position of the body (such as sitting on a stool or sitting with legs crossed on the floor, which is called the Lotus position):
2. Focus on the inflow and outflow of air streaming through the nostrils or of energy streaming in and out of a vital point, such as between the brows.
3. Focus attention on the rising and falling of the navel and the expansion and contraction of the abdomen.
4. Concentrate on a focal point, such as a candle flame or a mandala (a geometric meditation picture). Concentration during this step usually clears all other distractions from the mind.
5. Chant a mantra, the sacred syllables that harmonize energy and focus the mind. The three most commonly used mantras are "om," which stabilizes the body, "ah," which harmonizes energy, and "hum," which concentrates the spirit.

Beginning meditators should be advised that meditation must be practiced and that the "mind will be very uncooperative at first as the emotional mind fights against its own extinction by the higher forces of spiritual awareness" (Reid, 1994, p. 292). Meditation is viewed as an integral component of a person's daily routine.

Physical Exercise

Taoists modeled five physical exercises after five animals: the dragon, tiger, bear, eagle, and monkey. The movements of a particular animal are thought to stimulate a particular bodily organ. For healthy individuals, any of the exercises can be used to maintain a balanced physical and emotional state. If a specific problem exists, exercises directed to a specific organ are performed. Each exercise involves focusing on the image of the animal and miming the animal's movements. The moment the mind wanders, the exercise stops. For instance, for the ancient Chinese, the dragon was a mythical creature that symbolized the yang force of energy. The purpose of the dragon exercise (see Figure 8) is to instill the characteristics of the dragon, representing the fire element, into the mind and body. The physical effect of this exercise is to bring equilibrium to the heart and blood vessels and absorption in the small intestine. The other exercises are performed in a similar manner. The most important aspect of the exercises is the union of the body and mind; no benefit is obtained unless the body and mind are functioning in unison (Chang, 1986).

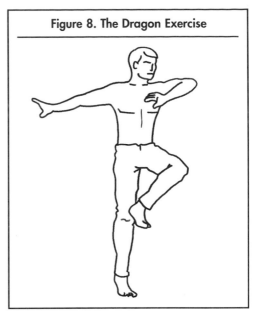

Figure 8. The Dragon Exercise

Healing Exercise

Healing exercise is divided into seven categories: therapeutic gymnastics, exercise therapy, mechanical therapy, Ch'i Kung (the Art of Breathing), An Mu (massage), nature's treatments (water showers, baths, air baths, and sun baths), and recreational exercise (Chang, 1985). Therapeutic gymnastics involve a series of special exercises that are chosen to assist in healing specific diseases or ailments. Each exercise series has a specific preparation, posture, exercise content, and number of repetitions. Emphasis is placed on the quality of the exercise rather than its quantity or variety. Exercise therapy is used to prevent as well as treat disease by improving the function of the heart and lungs. Tai chi is a form of exercise therapy that consists of slow, steady, smooth movements. The movements are flowing, intricate, and orderly and assist in developing grace, coordination, and balance. Tai chi is guided by peaceful, passive focusing and involves the whole body. Each movement strengthens and tones a different group of muscles and joints. Consistent practice makes joints more flexible and ligaments more elastic. Mechanical therapy involves the use of special exercise equipment, such as stationary bicycles, to restore function to the limbs and joints and to correct any deformities. Special wall-mounted wheels are used to promote flexibility and mobility of the arms and upper body. Qigong combines mental concentration with breathing exercises. It is designed to cultivate and nourish *qi*, or energy flow, within the body. Qigong often is used in the treatment of chronic diseases, such as depression, hypertension, and intestinal disorders. An Mu (massage) can be performed by the patient, a family member, or a practitioner. It is used to ease pain, stimulate blood and lymphatic circulation, increase muscle flexibility, accelerate digestion, reduce fatigue, and relax muscles. Nature's treatments, such as water showers or baths at various temperatures, can be invigorating or relaxing depending on the water temperature. Air baths and sun baths are believed to cleanse the lungs and skin. Recreational exercises include gardening and other hobbies that promote physical and psychological fitness.

Chee-gung Hand Balls

Since ancient times, Chinese calligraphers, painters, *chee-gung* healers, martial artists, and others whose livelihoods depended on strong, well-balanced hand energy and nimble fingers have used a simple method that is believed to balance internal energies, tone the tendons of the hands and arms, and increase the flow of energy to the palms and fingers. *Chee-gung* hand balls are two balls of equal size and weight made of steel, marble, agate, or jade. Jade is thought to be the best material because of its purported capacity to conduct and purify energy. Held in the palm of one hand, the balls are rolled in a circle by manipulating them with the fingers, counterclockwise in the right hand, clockwise in the left (see Figure 9). Beginners may experience clumsiness and may hear a loud "clack" of the balls as they are rotated. However, with practice, the balls will rotate smoothly, quietly, and quickly and produce a humming sound (Reid, 1994).

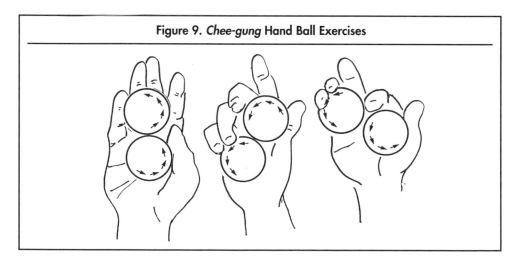

Figure 9. *Chee-gung* Hand Ball Exercises

Herbal Medicine

Herbal medicine is thought to predate acupuncture and is the primary form of treatment in some cultures. In the context of Chinese medicine, the term "herb" is used to describe any natural material of plant, animal, or mineral origin or any traditional or modern preparation of the natural materials short of preparing an isolated chemical (Xu, Zhu, & Xie, 1985). Chinese medicine contains a rich body of empirical knowledge of the use of medicinal plants for the treatment of various diseases (Qin & Xu, 1998). The traditional use of herbs is not based on their chemistry but rather selected to introduce certain qualities into the body and to balance or harmonize the dynamics that may be disrupted by illness or disease. Chinese herbs have been classified as medicines according to their origin and include (a) drugs originating from traditional medicine and ancient prescriptions, (b) drugs originating from folk prescriptions, and (c) drugs originating from Chinese herbs that have been modified and synthetically replicated (Xu et al.).

Chinese herbs are available in three forms. The most traditional are the raw materials themselves, which are boiled in water to make a beverage. The second form, a modern development, is the compression of the herbal substances into tablets or pills. The tablets or pills are viewed as more convenient to use, and the time required for and odor created from boiling herbs are eliminated. However, the tablets may be difficult to swallow and may require a large number to achieve the desired dose. Herbal extracts are provided in an eyedropper-type bottle in a concentrated form that is added to hot water and consumed as a tea. The extracts may be easier to consume and assimilate than tablets. Because they are in a liquid form, the extracts also allow combinations of herbal substances to be easily mixed, and a unique combination can be easily designed based on individual patient's needs (Collinge, 1996).

Herbal Treatments

In modern China, cancer is the leading cause of death (Parker, Tong, Bolden, & Wingo, 1997). Practitioners in China advocate a combination of Chinese and Western medicine as the optimal treatment for cancer, accompanied by diet, exercise, and lifestyle changes. The rationale for herbal use is twofold: to attack the cancer and to strengthen the patient's immune response. Chinese medicine uses more than 120 different herbs for cancer treatment, including a class of herbs called fu-zhen herbs (Collinge, 1996).

Few studies of the efficacy of traditional Chinese herbs in the treatment of various diseases have been conducted. In one study, Chinese herbs reduced or alleviated symptoms associated with asthma and allergies (But & Chang, 1996), and Chinese herbs have shown promise in the topical treatment of dermatologic disorders (Koo & Arain, 1998), but further empirical research is needed to determine the efficacy of Chinese herbal therapies.

Special Considerations

Although Chinese herbs can themselves be harmful (Macia, Navarro, Garcia-Nieto, & Garcia, 1995; Malik, 1995; Thomas, 1988), adverse drug interactions in patients using Chinese herbs are not widely recognized. For instance, Yu, Chan, and Sanderson (1997) found that concurrent use of warfarin and danshen, a Chinese herbal medicine widely used to treat cardiovascular disease, causes severe clotting abnormalities. Overanticoagulation and bleeding also were observed in patients who were receiving warfarin and had ingested the Chinese herb *Salvia miltiorrhizia* (Chan, 1998).

Aconitine-containing herbal preparations used for musculoskeletal pain were associated with two reported deaths (Dickens et al., 1994). Both patients had no history of cardiac disease and developed ventricular tachycardia, fibrillation, and cardiac arrest within 12 hours of ingesting the aconitine. Analysis of the herbal preparation confirmed the presence of aconitine in quantities in excess of the maximum recommended in the Chinese pharmacopoeia. Both patients were believed to have consumed an accidental overdose of aconitine, which has a narrow safety margin between therapeutic analgesic effect and its known cardiotoxic effect (Dickens et al.).

Every month, the U.S. Food and Drug Administration (FDA) receives dozens of reports of side effects caused by herbs. In June 1997, the FDA proposed regulations for the stimulant ma huang (ephedra), after it was linked to two deaths and implicated in 15 more (Bilger, 1997).

Acupuncture

Around 200 B.C., Jesuit missionaries returning from China reported the therapeutic use of needles and coined the term *acupuncture* from the Latin *acus*, meaning "needle," and *punctura*, meaning "pricking," to describe this treatment technique (Matsumoto, 1974). The origin of this method is unknown, although it has been suggested that cold weather forced the earliest physicians to develop a method of treatment that would not require the removal of clothing (Matsumoto). The techniques of acupuncture have been refined over the centuries and eventually spread to other Asian countries. During the 17th century, they were introduced in Europe (Reisser et al., 1987).

Western medicine began to take note of the practice of acupuncture in the mid-1970s. Bonica (1974) published a series of articles in *JAMA* reporting that thousands of successful surgical procedures were being performed in China using acupuncture anesthesia. In 1974, the Acupuncture Anesthesia Study Group of the

National Academy of Sciences observed 48 surgical procedures in 16 Chinese hospitals and concluded that acupuncture appeared to have promise as an anesthetic and as a treatment for pain control. A comprehensive literature search conducted by Astin, Marie, Pelletier, Hansen, and Haskell (1998) identified 25 surveys conducted from 1982–1995 that examined the practices and beliefs of conventional physicians with regard to five of the more prominent complementary therapies. Acupuncture had the highest rate of physician referral (43%) among the five therapies, and 51% of the physicians surveyed believed in its efficacy.

Goals of Acupuncture Therapy

The main goal of acupuncture therapy is to correct imbalances of yin and yang by stimulating specific points along the 12 meridians, thereby draining excesses of energy or restoring deficiencies. Approximately 365 points are first mapped on charts and then located on the patient using the landmarks of surface anatomy. The guidelines for selecting acupuncture points have evolved into a complex system based on laws that are believed to govern the five elements (Reisser et al., 1987).

The ancient Chinese believed that everything in the world represented components of yin and yang and belonged to one of five categories: wood, fire, earth, metal, and water. The five elements are believed to interact with one another in a specific manner. Each creates another (for example, wood creates fire) and is subjugated by a third (for example, metal subjugates wood). In addition, each of the five elements is associated with a particular color, season, direction, flavor, odor, and sound, and each organ in the body is related to one of the elements. The overall system often is represented by a diagram of interconnected circles. This diagram, which is reproduced in nearly all traditional acupuncture textbooks, is a road map of sorts for routing energies, as surplus ch'i is said to travel only in the direction of the arrows (see Figure 10).

Cohen, Kwok, and Cosic (1997) have offered a new explanation for how acupuncture works. They asserted that acupuncture may produce electrostimulation in accordance with the Seebeck effect, which refers to the production of a current when a temperature gradient exists across or between conductors. The acupuncture needles serve as conductors and produce internal currents, which are believed to have a therapeutic effect.

Other researchers believe that acupuncture excites receptors or nerve fibers in stimulated tissue and causes muscle contractions similar to those that occur from protracted exercise. Both exercise and acupuncture are thought to produce rhythmic discharges in nerve fibers and cause the release of endogenous opioids and oxytocin, which are essential to the induction of functional changes in various organ systems. Experimental and clinical evidence suggest that acupuncture may

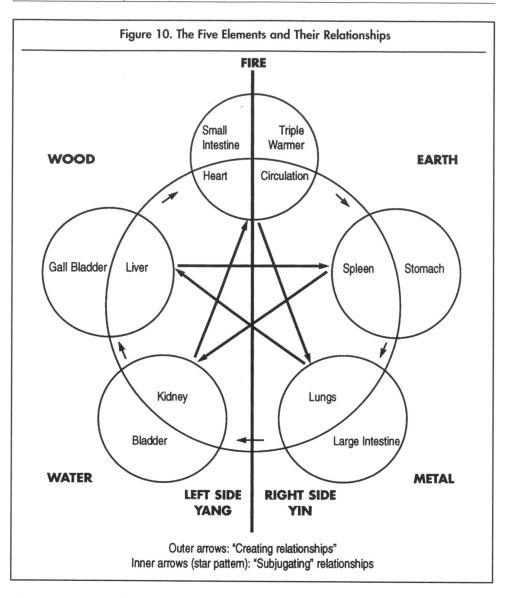

Figure 10. The Five Elements and Their Relationships

Outer arrows: "Creating relationships"
Inner arrows (star pattern): "Subjugating" relationships

affect the sympathetic system via mechanisms in the hypothalamic and brain stem levels and that the hypothalamic beta-endorphinergic system has inhibitory effects on the vasomotor center (Andersson & Lundeberg, 1995; Ulett, Han, & Han, 1998).

Acupuncture is viewed as a complete system of disease treatment. Potential indications for acupuncture include, but are not limited to, various diseases of the respiratory, ocular, gastrointestinal, and neuromuscular systems (Stux & Pomeranz, 1987). Some believe that acupuncture has a weak scientific foundation and recommend that rigorous controlled clinical trials be undertaken (Johnson, 1993).

The efficacy of acupuncture has been explored in a few studies. The incidence of postoperative nausea and vomiting was 35% in a group of patients receiving acupuncture and was found to be significantly less than the nausea and vomiting, which occurred in 65% of the placebo group in a randomized, double-blind study (al-Sadi, Newman, & Julious, 1997).

Moxibustion

Moxibustion treatment involves the burning of the herb moxa (mugwort) on an acupuncture point. Moxa is applied in the form of a fluffy material that is rolled up by the fingers into the size of a small pea, placed in position, and then lit, usually with an incense stick. It burns slowly, producing heat at the acupuncture point, and is removed by the practitioner when the patient feels it becoming hot, typically after a few seconds. Precautions must be taken to avoid burning the patient (Peterson, 1996). Moxibustion frequently is used with acupuncture, especially in rural China (Gu & Zhang, 1992).

Different kinds of moxa are available, and its effects are determined by factors such as its age, how tightly it is packed, how many applications are used on a given point, and its juxtaposition with needles. The moxa may be placed on a bed of salt, a piece of ginger, or a slice of garlic and then on the skin to introduce additional properties or influences into the acupuncture point (Collinge, 1996).

Acudetox

Acudetox refers to a specific addiction treatment approach in which acupuncture is used in conjunction with conventional methods of treating addictions to alcohol, drugs, and tobacco. The basic acudetox protocol consists of the placement of five acupuncture needles in each ear at specified sites, which are called shen, men, liver, lung, kidney, and sympathetic. Additional points may be targeted in the ear, head, or arms to treat associated conditions, such as headache, depression, or insomnia. Approximately 300 acudetox programs exist in the United States, and most programs involve the administration of daily acudetox treatment for two weeks, then three times a week for four weeks (Schulte, 1996). Treatment usually is given in a group setting, with patients sitting quietly with the acupuncture needles in place for 30–40 minutes. The success of the acudetox treatment has prompted several prison systems to use this approach, and first-time drug offenders in Dade County, FL, are offered acudetox treatment as an alternative to incarceration. Estimates indicate that acudetox costs approximately $750 per year per patient, while a year of incarceration costs $22,000 or more (Schulte).

Special Considerations

Many studies of acupuncture treatment are seriously flawed by methodological problems. Poor design, inadequate measures and statistical analysis, lack of follow-up data, and substandard treatment are common.

A major problem is the definition of an appropriate placebo control (Harden, 1994; Vincent & Lewith, 1995). The lack of uniformity in research design and the lack of controlled studies limit the conclusions that can be made about the effectiveness of acupuncture as a treatment modality (Ernst & White, 1997). Reisser et al. (1987) observed that acupuncture does, indeed, relieve pain to varying degrees in large numbers of patients with a wide variety of disorders. However, physicians cannot easily predict which patients will respond most favorably. The duration of pain relief often varies and can range from transient to permanent. Pain from cancer or trauma usually does not improve with acupuncture, while dental pain tends to respond more consistently. Cultural conditioning, the belief that acupuncture will work, friendly surroundings, and the patient's mood also appear to affect results.

Adverse effects and complications secondary to acupuncture have been reported (see Figure 11). The most frequent complication is the vasovagal episode (Peterson, 1996). Other, more serious, complications and adverse effects have been associated with acupuncture, including pneumothorax following acupuncture (Olusanya & Mansuri, 1997; Vilke & Wulfert, 1997), drop foot as a result of direct injury to the common peroneal nerve by an acupuncture needle (Sobel, Huang, & Wieting, 1997), motor and sensory impairment caused by migration of an acupuncture needle into the medulla oblongata (Abumi, Anbo, & Kaneda, 1996), a fatal cardiac tamponade after acupuncture through a congenital sternal foramen (Halvorsen, Anda, Naess, & Levang, 1995), and endocarditis (Lee & McIllwain, 1985; Scheel, Sundsfjord, Lunde, & Andersen, 1992). A 29-year-old man reportedly died from a severe asthmatic attack while undergoing acupuncture and moxibustion treatment (Ogata, Kitamura, Kubo, & Nakasono, 1992).

Figure 11. Complications Associated With Acupuncture
Vasovagal episodes
Pneumothorax
Peroneal nerve injury
Motor and sensory impairment
Cardiac tamponade
Otitis externa
Perichondritis
Hepatitis B

Otitis externa and perichondritis have occurred with auricular acupuncture, and these complications are difficult to eradicate because of the poor vascularization of cartilage (Carron, Epstein, & Grand, 1974). Reports of hepatitis B associated with an acupuncture clinic using improperly sterilized reusable needles also have been published ("Hepatitis B," 1992). Baldry (1993) noted that while acupuncture is a fairly low-risk procedure, the practice of acupuncture needs tighter safeguards. Experienced practitioners who carefully screen patients and use disposable needles or proper sterilization procedures for reusable needles should be consulted for acupuncture therapy.

Massage (Acupressure, Shiatsu)

Acupressure and shiatsu sometimes are described as acupuncture without needles. Shiatsu is viewed as the Japanese version of acupressure; *shi* means "finger" and *atsu* means "pressure" (Schindler, 1997). The geography of points and meridians, similar to those used for acupuncture, is used to guide the application of finger or palm pressure rather than the insertion of needles. The aims of therapy also are similar in terms of stimulating points and influencing the flow of ch'i through the meridians. Acupressure is applied by the fingertips to create gentle but firm pressure. Generally, pressure is held for two to five minutes at each point; it is believed that an experienced practitioner can feel a slight pulse when compressing a point. During the process of holding and releasing the various pressure points during a single session, which usually lasts about an hour, the patient typically becomes very calm as the body secretes endorphins and enkephalins, which are viewed as relaxation hormones that assist the body in healing itself (Maxwell, 1997). Further details of these therapies are discussed in Chapter 4, "Manual Healing Methods."

Special Considerations

In China, Western medicine and traditional medicine are practiced together at every level of the healthcare system. Traditional treatments account for approximately 40% of all health care delivered in China (Hesketh & Zhu, 1997), and health care is provided with an emphasis on prevention to nearly all of its citizens (Hesketh & Wei, 1997). Current research priorities in China include randomized, controlled trials of common treatments, such as herbal remedies, acupuncture, acupressure, massage, and moxibustion, to scientifically verify their efficacy. Healthcare practitioners in China envision that their integrated approach of healthcare delivery will be adopted in other countries in the near future (Hesketh & Zhu). Journal articles have been published to educate primary-care providers about the basic principles of acupuncture, indications, and considerations for appropriate patient selection (Peterson, 1996; Urba, 1996).

An estimated 9–12 million patient visits per year are made to practitioners of Chinese medicine in the United States, most seeking acupuncture for treatment of pain symptoms after experiencing unsatisfactory results with Western medicine (Lytle, 1993). The United States has 9,000–10,000 practitioners of acupuncture and 35 schools of Chinese medicine that train nonphysician practitioners. In 1973, Nevada became the first state to license nonphysician practitioners of acupuncture. Twenty-three states restrict the practice of acupuncture to physicians only, while the remainder have varying degrees of regulation for nonphysicians (Collinge, 1996).

Chinese medicine often is used in conjunction with other forms of medicine, including Western medicine, allopathy, or osteopathy. Chiropractors sometimes are trained in acupuncture, and Chinese medicine is a specialty of many naturopaths, who use it along with other forms of natural medicine.

Costs of Traditional Oriental Medicine

Patient fees for traditional Oriental medicine basically are for treatment time in the practitioner's office and for herbal remedies. Initial sessions with nonphysician practitioners may range from $50 to $100 (more for physicians), and follow-up sessions typically cost less. The number of treatment sessions varies depending on the nature of the ailment. A typical course of acupuncture treatment may be once or twice a week for several weeks, with treatments spaced further apart as time progresses. More difficult chronic illnesses may require treatment over several months. The cost of herbs varies widely, ranging anywhere from $10 to $50 or more per month (Collinge, 1996).

Insurance companies differ in their coverage, and a variety of factors influence these differences, including state regulations, licensure of the practitioner, and whether medical supervision is required. Some states authorize Medicaid to pay for alcohol and substance abuse treatment by licensed or certified acupuncturists (Collinge, 1996). In 1996, the U.S. Government recognized acupuncture needles as medical devices; it is expected that nongovernmental insurers will be more likely to cover acupuncture treatment in the future ("Housecalls," 1997).

Ballegaard, Norrelund, and Smith (1996) explored the cost-benefit of traditional Chinese therapies. Sixty-nine patients with severe angina pectoris received acupuncture and shiatsu and were followed for two years. Invasive treatment was postponed in 61% of the patients because of clinical improvement, and the annual number of in-hospital days was reduced by 90%. The economic savings was estimated to be $12,000 per patient.

Summary

Naturopathy, homeopathy, environmental medicine, and folk medicine are a few of many types of alternative medical systems that have been used by patients in the treatment of various disorders. Although a paucity of large, randomized, controlled trials have evaluated the efficacy of these treatments, there is sufficient evidence to suggest that many of these therapies can produce objective as well as subjective benefit in selected groups of patients. In view of the increasing popularity of complementary medicine among patients and general practitioners, there is now an urgent need to conduct high-quality research to determine how, or whether, these therapies may be interwoven with the more orthodox treatments currently available (Lewith & Watkins, 1996).

References

Abumi, K., Anbo, H., & Kaneda, K. (1996). Migration of an acupuncture needle into the medulla oblongata. *European Spine Journal, 5*(2), 137–139.

Achterberg, J. (1985). *Imagery in healing: Shamanism and modern medicine.* Boston: Shambhala.

Adler, S.R. (1995). Refugee stress and folk belief: Hmong sudden deaths. *Social Science and Medicine, 40,* 1623–1629.

Albertson, E. (1996). The facts of fasting. *American Health: Fitness of Body and Mind, 15*(6), 64–65.

al-Sadi, M., Newman, B., & Julious, S.A. (1997). Acupuncture in the prevention of postoperative nausea and vomiting. *Anaesthesia, 52,* 658–661.

Ancelet, B.J. (1994). *Cajun and Creole folktales. The French oral tradition of south Louisiana.* Jackson, MS: University Press of Mississippi.

Andersson, S., & Lundeberg, T. (1995). Acupuncture—From empiricism to science: Functional background to acupuncture effects in pain and disease. *Medical Hypotheses, 45,* 271–281.

Anthroposophic Press. (1997). *Rudolf Steiner and anthroposophy* [Online]. Available: www.anthropress.org/press/SteinerProf.html [1999, April 6].

Applewhite, S.L. (1995). Curanderismo: Demystifying the health beliefs and practices of elderly Mexican Americans. *Health and Social Work, 20,* 247–253.

Astin, J.A., Marie, A., Pelletier, K.R., Hansen, E., & Haskell, W.L. (1998). A review of the incorporation of complementary and alternative medicine by mainstream physicians. *Archives of Internal Medicine, 158,* 2303–2310.

Baer, H.A. (1992). The potential rejuvenation of American naturopathy as a consequence of the holistic health movement. *Medical Anthropology, 13,* 369–383.

Baker, J.P. (1992). The shamanic dimensions of childbirth. *Pre- and Peri-Natal Psychology Journal, 7*(1), 5–21.

Baldry, P. (1993). Complementary medicine. The practice of acupuncture needs tighter safeguards. *British Medical Journal, 307,* 326.

Ballegaard, S., Norrelund, S., & Smith, D.F. (1996). Cost-benefit of combined use of acupuncture, shiatsu and lifestyle adjustment fot treatment of patients with severe angina pectoris. *Acupuncture and Electro-Therapeutics Research, 21*(3–4), 187–197.

Bao, K. (1992). Comments on nomenclature in traditional Chinese medicine. *American Journal of Chinese Medicine, 20*(2), 191–194.

Bayly, G.R., Braithwaite, R.A., Sheehan, T.M., Dyer, N.H., Grimley, C., & Ferner, R.E. (1995). Lead poisoning from Asian traditional remedies in the West Midlands—Report of a series of five cases. *Human and Experimental Toxicology, 14*(1), 24–28.

Begley, S.S. (1994). Tibetan Buddhist medicine: A transcultural nursing experience. *Journal of Holistic Nursing, 12,* 323–342.

Berry, R.G., & Collymore, V.A. (1993). Otitis externa and facial cellulitis from Oriental ear cleaners. *Western Journal of Medicine, 158,* 536.

Bilger, B. (1997). Nature's pharmacy. *Hippocrates: Health and Medicine for Physicians, 11*(11), 20–24.

Bonica, J.J. (1974). Therapeutic acupuncture in the People's Republic of China: Implications for American medicine. *JAMA, 228,* 1544–1551.

Booth, B. (1994). Complementary medicine. Naturopathy. *Nursing Times, 90*(7), 44–46.

Bostrom, H., & Rossner, S. (1990). Quality of alternative medicine: Complications and avoidable death. *Quality Assurance in Health Care, 2,* 111–117.

Bouchager, F. (1990). Alternative medicine: A general approach to the French situation. *Complementary Medicine Research, 4,* 4–8.

Brewer, J.A., & Bonalumi, N.M. (1995). Cultural diversity in the emergency department: Health care beliefs and practices among the Pennsylvania Amish. *Journal of Emergency Nursing, 21,* 494–497.

Brooks, S.M., Gochfeld, M., Herzstein, J., Schenker, M., & Jackson, R. (Eds.). (1995). *Environmental medicine: Principles and practice.* St. Louis: Mosby.

Broussard, B.A., Sugarman, J.R., Bachman-Carter, K., Booth, K., Stephenson, L., Strauss, K., & Gohdes, D. (1995). Toward comprehensive obesity prevention programs in Native American communities. *Obesity Research, 3*(Suppl. 2), 289–297.

Buccalo, S. (1997). Window on another world: An "English" nurse looks at the Amish culture and their health care beliefs. *Journal of Multicultural Nursing and Health, 3*(2), 53–58.

But, P., & Chang, C. (1996). Chinese herbal medicine in the treatment of asthma and allergies. *Clinical Reviews in Allergy and Immunology, 14*(3), 253–269.

Campbell, J. (1983). *The way of animal powers.* London: Summerfield Press.

Campinha-Bacote, J. (1992). Voodoo illness. *Perspectives in Psychiatric Care, 28*(1), 11–19.

Campinha-Bacote, J. (1998). African Americans. In L. Purnell & B. Paulanka (Eds.), *Transcultural health care: A culturally competent approach.* Philadelphia: F.A. Davis Co.

Carron, H., Epstein, B.S., & Grand, B. (1974). Complications of acupuncture. *JAMA, 228,* 1553–1556.

Castilla, E.E., & Adams, J. (1996). Genealogical information and the structure of rural Latin-American populations: Reality and fantasy. *Human Heredity, 46,* 241–255.

Cates, P. (1996). Secret ceremony. *Nursing96, 26*(8), 72.

Cavender, A. (1996). Local unorthodox healers of cancer in the Appalachian south. *Journal of Community Health, 21,* 359–374.

Cerrato, P.L. (1989). How safe are modified fasts? *RN, 52*(11), 79–81.

Chan, T.Y. (1998). Drug interactions as a cause of overanticoagulation and bleedings in Chinese patients receiving warfarin. *International Journal of Clinical Pharmacology Therapy, 36,* 403–405.

Chang, E.C. (Trans.). (1985). *Knocking at the gate of life and other healing exercises from China. The official handbook of the People's Republic of China.* Emmaus, PA: Rodale Press.

Chang, S.T. (1986). *The complete system of self-healing. Internal exercises.* San Francisco: Tao Publishing.

Cheon-Klessig, Y., Camilleri, D.D., Mc Elmurry, B.J., & Ohlson, V.M. (1988). Folk medicine in the health practice of Hmong refugees. *Western Journal of Nursing Research, 10,* 647–660.

Cherry, B., & Giger, J.N. (1995). African-Americans. In J.N. Giger & R.E. Davidhizar (Eds.), *Transcultural nursing: Assessment and intervention* (pp. 165–203). St. Louis: Mosby.

Chopra, D. (1991). *Perfect health. The complete mind/body guide.* New York: Harmony Books.

Chowka, P.B. (1996). *Utah becomes the ninth state to license naturopathic medicine* [Online]. Available: www.anma.net [1997, November 12].

Chowka, P.B. (1997). *What is naturopathic medicine? The history and practice in North America* [Online]. Available: www.anma.net [1997, November 12].

Cohen, K. (1998). Native American medicine. *Alternative Therapies in Health and Medicine, 4*(6), 45–57.

Cohen, M., Kwok, G., & Cosic, I. (1997). Acupuncture needles and the Seebeck effect: Do temperature gradients produce electrostimulation? *Acupuncture and Electro-Therapeutics Research, 22*(1), 9–15.

Collinge, W. (1996). *The American Holistic Health Association complete guide to alternative medicine.* New York: Warner Books, Inc.

Cook, L.S., & de Mange, B.P. (1995). Gaining access to Native American cultures by non-Native American nursing researchers. *Nursing Forum, 30*(1), 5–10.

Cooper, R.A., & Stoflet, S.J. (1996). Trends in the education and practice of alternative medicine clinicians. *Health Affairs, 15*(3), 226–238.

Cordes, D.H., Rea, D.F., Rea, J.L., & Peate, W.F. (1996). Occupational and environmental medicine in preventionist residency training programs. *Journal of Occupational and Environmental Medicine, 38,* 615–618.

Cowan, T. (1993). *Fired in the head. Shamanism and the Celtic spirit.* San Francisco: HaperSanFrancisco.

Cummings, S., & Ullman, D. (1997). *Everybody's guide to homeopathic medicines* (2nd ed.). Los Angeles: Tarcher.

Damery, P. (1997). Shamanic states in our lives and in analytic practice. In D.F. Sandner & S.H. Wong (Eds.), *The sacred heritage: The influence of shamanism on analytical psychology* (pp. 71–77). New York: Routledge.

Daniels, G.J., & McCabe, P. (1994). Nursing diagnosis and natural therapies. A symbiotic relationship. *Journal of Holistic Nursing, 12*(2), 184–192.

Dickens, P., Tai, Y.T., But, P.P., Tomlinson, B., Ng, H.K., & Yan, K.W. (1994). Fatal accidental aconitine poisoning following ingestion of Chinese herbal medicine: A report of two cases. *Forensic Science International, 67,* 55–58.

Dobkin de Rios, M., & Winkelman, M. (1989). Shamanism and altered states of consciousness: An introduction. *Journal of Psychoactive Drugs, 21*(1), 1–7.

Donden, Y. (1986). *Health through balance. An introduction to Tibetan medicine.* Ithaca, NY: Snow Lion Publications.

Dunbabin, D.W., Tallis, G.A., Popplewell, P.Y., & Lee, R.A. (1992). Lead poisoning from Indian herbal medicine (Ayurveda). *Medical Journal of Australia, 157,* 835–836.

Edelstein, S.J., & Stevenson, I. (1983). Sickle cell anaemia and reincarnation beliefs in Nigeria. *Lancet, 2*(8359), 1140.

Ellis, J.L., & Campos-Outcalt, D. (1994). Cardiovascular disease risk factors in Native Americans: A literature review. *American Journal of Preventive Medicine, 10,* 295–307.

Emmett, E.A. (1996). What is the strategic value of occupational and environmental medicine? Observations from the United States and Australia. *Journal of Occupational and Environmental Medicine, 28,* 1124–1134.

Ernst, E. (1996). Towards quality in complementary health care: Is the German "Heilpraktiker" a model for complementary practitioners? *International Journal for Quality in Health Care, 8*(2), 187–190.

Ernst, E., & Kaptchuk, T.J. (1996). Homeopathy revisited. *Archives of Internal Medicine, 156,* 2162–2164.

Ernst, E., & Pittler, M.H. (1998). Efficacy of homeopathic arnica: A systematic review of placebo-controlled clinical trials. *Archives of Surgery, 133,* 1187–1190.

Ernst, E., & White, A.R. (1997). A review of problems in clinical acupuncture research. *American Journal of Chinese Medicine, 25*(1), 3–11.

Exley, C., Sim, J., Reid, N., Jackson, S., & West, N. (1996). Attitudes and beliefs within the Sikh community regarding organ donation: A pilot study. *Social Science and Medicine, 43,* 23–28.

Finckh, E. (1981). Tibetan medicine: Theory and practice. *American Journal of Chinese Medicine, 9,* 259–267.

Foundation for Shamanic Studies. (1997). *Frequently asked questions about FSS and shamanism* [Online]. Available: www.shamanism.org/faq.html [1999, April 7].

Fulder, S. (1987). *The Tao of medicine. Oriental remedies and the pharmacology of harmony.* Rochester, VT: Destiny Books.

Fye, W.B. (1986). Nitroglycerine: A homeopathic remedy. *Circulation, 73,* 21–29.

Garrett, J.T., & Garrett, M. (1996). *Medicine of the Cherokee. The way of right relationship.* Santa Fe, NM: Bear & Co.

Gerson, S. (1993). *Ayurveda: The ancient Indian healing art.* Rockport, MA: Element Books.

Gervais, K.G. (1996). Providing culturally competent health care to Hmong patients. *Minnesota Medicine, 79*(5), 49–51.

Giger, J.N., & Davidhizar, R.E. (1995). Environmental control. In J.N. Giger & R.E. Davidhizar (Eds.), *Transcultural nursing: Assessment and intervention* (pp. 113–125). St. Louis: Mosby.

Gillum, R.F. (1995). The epidemiology of stroke in Native Americans. *Stroke, 26,* 514–521.

Giovannucci, E., Rimm, E.B., Colditz, G.A., Stampfer, M.J., Ascherio, A., Chute, C.C., & Willett, W.C. (1993). A prospective study of dietary fat and risk of prostate cancer. *Journal of the National Cancer Institute, 85,* 1571–1579.

Glisson, J., Crawford, R., & Street, S. (1999). Review, critique, and guidelines for the use of herbs and homeopathy. *Nurse Practitioner, 24*(4), 44–46, 53, 60, 62.

Gohel, D., & Dave, T. (1991). Ayurvedic drugs. No more innocent. *Journal of the Association of Physicians in India, 39,* 294.

Goldberg, B. (1982). *Past lives, future lives.* New York: Ballantine Books.

Goldbohm, R.A., van den Brandt, P.A, van't Veer, P., Brants, A.M., Dorant, E., Sturmans, F., & Hermus, R.J.J. (1994). A prospective cohort study on the relation between meat consumption and the risk of colon cancer. *Cancer Research, 54,* 718–723.

Goldstein, M.S., & Glik, D. (1998). Use of and satisfaction with homeopathy in a patient population. *Alternative Therapies in Health and Medicine, 4*(2), 60–65.

Gu, J.C., & Zhang, L.M. (1992). Acupuncture and moxibustion in primary health care in rural China. *World Health Forum, 13*(1), 51.

Gunn, S.W. (1995). Totemic medicine among the American Indians of the northwest coast. *Patient Education and Counseling, 26*(1–3), 159–167.

Gustafson, M.B. (1989). Western voodoo: Providing mental health care to Haitian refugees. *Journal of Psychosocial Nursing and Mental Health Services, 27*(1), 30–31.

Halper, J., & Berger, L.R. (1981). Naturopaths and childhood immunizations: Heterodoxy among the unorthodox. *Pediatrics, 68,* 407–410.

Halvorsen, T.B., Anda, S.S., Naess, A.B., & Levang, O.W. (1995). Fatal cardiac tamponade after acupuncture through congenital sternal foramen. *Lancet, 345*(8958), 1175.

Hanley, C.E. (1995). Navajo Indians. In J.N. Giger & R.E. Davidhizar (Eds.), *Transcultural nursing: Assessment and intervention* (pp. 237–260). St. Louis: Mosby.

Harden, R.N. (1994). The pitfalls of clinical acupuncture research: Can east satisfy west? *Arthritis Care and Research, 7*(3), 115–117.

Harner, M. (1990). *The way of the shaman.* New York: HarperCollins.

Health and Human Services Dept. (1992). *Alternative medicine. Expanding medical horizons.* Washington, DC: U.S. Government Printing Office.

Hepatitis B associated with an acupuncture clinic. (1992, November 27). *Communicable Disease Report. CDR Weekly, 2*(48), 219.

Hesketh, T., & Wei, X.Z. (1997). Health in China. From Mao to market reform. *British Medical Journal, 314,* 1543–1545.

Hesketh, T., & Zhu, W.X. (1997). Health in China. Traditional Chinese medicine: One country, two systems. *British Medical Journal, 315,* 115–117.

Hollifield, S.C. (1998). *Calm Spirit magazine* [Online]. Available: http://ourworld.compuserve .com/homepages/CalmSpirit/CalmPage.htm [1999, April 7].

Housecalls. (1997). *Hippocrates: Health and Medicine for Physicians, 11*(11), 32.

Hudson, T. (1993). Escharotic treatment for cervical dysplasia and carcinoma. *Journal of Naturopathic Medicine, 4*(1), 23–30.

Hudson, T., & Standish, L. (1993). *Clinical and endocrinologic effects of a menopausal formula.* Paper presented at the American Association of Naturopathic Physicians Convention, Portland, OR.

Indian Health Service. (1997a). *Comprehensive health care program for American Indians and Alaska Natives: IHS accomplishments* [Online]. Available: www.ihs.gov/nonmedicalprograms/ profiles/profileaccomp.asp [1999, April 6].

Indian Health Service. (1997b). *Comprehensive health care program for American Indians and Alaska Natives: Indian health today* [Online]. Available: www.ihs.gov/nonmedicalprograms/ profiles/profileihtoday.asp [1999, April 6].

Jacobs, J., Chapman, E.H., & Crothers, D. (1998). Patient characteristics and practice patterns of physicians using homeopathy. *Archives of Family Medicine, 7,* 537–540.

Jacobs, J., Jiminez, L.M., Gloyd, S.S., Gale, J.L., & Crothers, D. (1994). Treatment of childhood diarrhea with homeopathic medicines: A randomized clinical trial in Nicaragua. *Pediatrics, 93,* 719–725.

Johnson, I.S. (1993). Complementary medicine. Acupuncture has weak scientific foundations. *British Medical Journal, 307,* 624.

Jue, R.W. (1996). Past-life therapy. In B.W. Scotton, A.B. Chinen, & J.R. Battista (Eds.), *Textbook of transpersonal psychiatry and psychology* (pp. 377–387). New York: Basic Books.

Jun, J.B., Min, P.K., Kim, D.W., Chung, S.L., & Lee, K.H. (1997). Cutaneous nodular reaction to oral mercury. *Journal of the American Academy of Dermatology, 37,* 131–133.

Kalweit, H. (1988). *Dreamtime and inner space: The world of the shaman.* Boston: Shambhala.

Keegan, L. (1996). Use of alternative therapies among Mexican Americans in the Texas Rio Grande Valley. *Journal of Holistic Nursing, 14,* 277–294.

Kilbourne, E.M. (1994). Overview of environmental medicine. In L. Rosenstock & M.R. Cullen (Eds.), *Textbook of clinical occupational and environmental medicine* (pp. 41–47). Philadelphia: Saunders.

King, F.J. (1996). Homeopathy for the holistic nurse: Classical vs. contemporary homeopathy. *Beginnings, 16*(8), 9.

Koo, J., & Arain, S. (1998). Traditional Chinese medicine for the treatment of dermatologic disorders. *Archives of Dermatology, 134,* 1388–1393.

Kuipers, J. (1995). Mexican Americans. In J.N. Giger & R.E. Davidhizar (Eds.), *Transcultural nursing: Assessment and intervention* (pp. 205–234). St. Louis: Mosby.

Kushi, M. (1992). *Other dimensions: Exploring the unexplained.* Garden City Park, NY: Avery Publishing Group.

Lad, V.D. (1984). *Ayurveda: The science of self-healing: A practical guide.* Santa Fe, NM: Lotus Press.

Lee, R.J., & McIllwain, J.C. (1985). Subacute bacterial endocarditis following ear acupuncture. *International Journal of Cardiology, 7,* 62–63.

Leland, J., & Power, C. (1997, October 20). Deepak's instant karma. *Newsweek,* pp. 52–58.

LeMaster, P.L., & Connell, C.M. (1994). Health education interventions among Native Americans: A review and analysis. *Health Education Quarterly, 21,* 521–538.

Lewith, G.T., & Watkins, A.D. (1996). Unconventional therapies in asthma: An overview. *Allergy, 51,* 761–769.

Linde, K., & Melchart, D. (1998).Randomized controlled trials of individualized homeopathy: A state-of-the-art review. *Journal of Alternative and Complementary Medicine, 4,* 371–388.

Lytle, C.D. (1993). *An overview of acupuncture.* Rockville, MD: Public Health Service, Food and Drug Administration, Centers for Devices and Radiological Health.

Macia, M., Navarro, J., Garcia-Nieto, V., & Garcia, J. (1995). Chinese herbs can themselves be harmful. *Arthritis and Rheumatism, 39,* 354–355.

Malik, T. (1995). The safety of herbal medicine. *Alternative Therapies in Health and Medicine, 1*(4), 27–28.

Marriott, J. (1984). Hypnotic regression and past lives therapy: Fantasy or reality? *Australian Journal of Hypnotherapy and Hypnosis, 5*(2), 65–72.

Matsumoto, T. (1974). *Acupuncture for physicians.* Springfield, IL: Charles C. Thomas.

Maxwell, J. (1997). The gentle power of acupressure. *RN, 60*(4), 53–56.

McWhorter, J.H. (1996). Spicebush. A Cherokee remedy for the measles. *North Carolina Medical Journal, 57,* 306.

Mehl-Madrona, L.E. (1999). Native American medicine in the treatment of chronic illness: Developing an integrated program and evaluating its effectiveness. *Alternative Therapies in Health and Medicine, 5*(1), 36–44.

Moody, R.A. (1990). *Coming back. A psychiatrist explores past-life journeys.* New York: Bantam Books.

Moore, M.P. (1997). Unraveling the mysteries of environmental medicine. *Minnesota Medicine, 80*(1), 12–20.

Mosek, A., & Korczyn, A.D. (1996). Fasting and headache. *Headache Quarterly, Current Treatment and Research, 7,* 215–217.

Mosihuzzaman, M., Nahar, N., Ali, L., Rokeya, B., Khan, A.K., Nur-E-Alam, M., & Nandi, R.P. (1994). Hypoglycemic effects of three plants from eastern Himalayan belt. *Diabetes Research, 26,* 127–138.

Muneta, B., Newman, J., Wetterall, S., & Stevenson, J. (1993). Diabetes and associated risk factors among Native Americans. *Diabetes Care, 16,* 1619–1620.

Murray, M., & Pizzorno, J. (1991). *The encyclopedia of natural medicine.* Rocklin, CA: Prima Publishing.

National Native American AIDS Prevention Center. (1997). *June 1998 AIDS and HIV statistics for AI/AN now available* [Online]. Available: www.nnaapc.org [1999, April 6].

Ogata, M., Kitamura, O., Kubo, S., & Nakasono, I. (1992). An asthmatic death while under Chinese acupuncture and moxibustion treatment. *American Journal of Forensic Medicine and Pathology, 13,* 338–341.

Oliver, M.R., Van Voorhis, W.C., Boeckh, M., Mattson, D., & Bowden, R.A. (1996). Hepatic mucormycosis in a bone marrow transplant recipient who ingested naturopathic medicine. *Clinical Infectious Diseases, 22,* 521–524.

Olusanya, O., & Mansuri, I. (1997). Pneumothorax following acupuncture. *Journal of the American Board of Family Practice, 10,* 296–297.

Onwubalili, J.K. (1983). Sickle-cell anaemia: An explanation for the ancient myth of reincarnation in Nigeria. *Lancet, 2*(8348), 503–505.

Oriol, M.D. (1995). Cajun traditions and their impact on health care. *Journal of Cultural Diversity, 2*(1), 27–30.

Ornish, D. (1990). *Dr. Dean Ornish's program for reversing heart disease.* New York: Random House.

Ornish, D., Brown, S.E., Scherwitz, L.W., Billings, J.H., Armstrong, W.T., Ports, T.A., McLanahan, S.M., Kirkeeide, R.L., Brand, R.J., & Gould, K.L. (1990). Can lifestyle changes reverse coronary artery disease? *Lancet, 336*(8708), 129–132.

Ortner, S.B. (1995). The case of the disappearing shamans, or no individualism, no relationalism. *Ethos, 23,* 355–390.

Paranjpe, P., & Kulkarni, P.H. (1995). Comparative efficacy of four Ayurvedic formulations in the treatment of acne vulgaris: A double-blind randomized placebo-controlled clinical evaluation. *Journal of Ethnopharmacology, 49*(3), 127–132.

Parish, R.A., McIntire, S., & Heimbach, D.M. (1987). Garlic burns: A naturopathic remedy gone awry. *Pediatric Emergency Care, 3,* 258–260.

Parker, S.L., Tong, T., Bolden, S., & Wingo, P.A. (1997). Cancer statistics, 1997. *CA: A Cancer Journal for Clinicians, 47,* 5–27.

Peterson, J.R. (1996). Acupuncture in the 1990s. A review for the primary care physician. *Archives of Family Medicine, 5,* 237–240.

Prasad, M.L., Parry, P., & Chan, C. (1993). Ayurvedic agents produce differential effects on murine and human melanoma cells in vitro. *Nutrition and Cancer, 20,* 79–86.

Prpic-Majic, D., Pizent, A., Jurasovic, J., Pongracic, J., & Restek-Samarzija, N. (1996). Lead poisoning associated with the use of Ayurvedic metal-mineral tonics. *Journal of Toxicology Clinical Toxicology, 34,* 417–423.

Purnell, L., & Counts, M. (1998). Appalachians. In L. Purnell & B. Paulanka (Eds.), *Transcultural health care* (pp. 107–136). Philadelphia: F.A. Davis Co.

Qin, G.W., & Xu, R.S. (1998). Recent advances on bioactive natural products from Chinese medicinal plants. *Medical Research Reviews, 18,* 375–382.

Quillin, P. (1996). *Amish folk medicine.* Canton, OH: The Leader Company, Inc.

Ramster, P. (1994). Past lives and hypnosis. *Australian Journal of Clinical Hypnotherapy and Hypnosis, 15*(2), 67–91.

Rapgay, L. (1986). A guide to Tibetan medical urinalysis. *Acupuncture and Electro-Therapeutics Research, 11*(1), 25–43.

Redfield, J. (1993). *The Celestine prophecy: An adventure.* New York: Warner Books.

Reed, E. (1990). *Wet graves, hoodoo men and sharp cats. The history of pharmacy in Louisiana from the very beginning.* Baton Rouge, LA: Ed Reed Organization.

Reid, D. (1994). *The complete book of Chinese health and healing. Guarding the three treasures.* Boston: Shambhala.

Reilly, D., Taylor, M.A., Beattie, N.G., Campbell, J.H., McSharry, C., Atchison, T.C., Carter, R., & Stevenson, R.D. (1994). Is evidence for homeopathy reproducible? *Lancet, 344*(8937), 1601–1606.

Reisser, P.C., Reisser, T.K., & Weldon, J. (1987). *New age medicine.* Downers Grove, IL: Intervarsity Press.

Rioux, D. (1996). Shamanic healing techniques: Toward holistic addiction counseling. *Alcoholism Treatment Quarterly, 14*(1), 59–69.

Risser, A.L., & Mazur, L.J. (1995). Use of folk remedies in a Hispanic population. *Archives of Pediatrics and Adolescent Medicine, 149,* 978–981.

Rosenstock, L., & Cullen, M.R. (1994). *Textbook of clinical occupational and environmental medicine.* Philadelphia: Saunders.

Ruiz, P. (1985). Cultural barriers to effective medical care among Hispanic-American patients. *Annual Review of Medicine, 36,* 63–71.

Ryan, M. (1997). Efficacy of the Tibetan treatment for arthritis. *Social Science and Medicine, 44,* 535–539.

Sanchez, T.R., Plawecki, J.A., & Plawecki, H.M. (1996). The delivery of culturally sensitive health care to Native Americans. *Journal of Holistic Nursing, 14,* 295–307.

Scheel, O., Sundsfjord, A., Lunde, P., & Andersen, B.M. (1992). Endocarditis after acupuncture and injection. *JAMA, 267,* 56.

Schindler, M. (1997, November-December). Natural stress relief. *Natural Health,* pp. 113–132.

Schulte, E. (1996). Acupuncture: Where east meets west. *RN, 59*(10), 55–57.

Shadick, K.M. (1993). Development of a transcultural health education program for the Hmong. *Clinical Nurse Specialist, 7*(2), 48–53.

Sharma, R.R. (1986). Homeopathy today: A scientific appraisal. *British Homeopathic Journal, 75,* 231–236.

Simpson, J.J., Donaldson, I., & Davies, W.E. (1998). Use of homeopathy in the treatment of tinnitus. *Brisith Journal of Audiology, 32,* 227–233.

Skaer, T.L., Robison, L.M., Sclar, D.A., & Harding, G.H. (1996). Utilization of curanderos among foreign born Mexican-American women attending migrant health clinics. *Journal of Cultural Diversity, 3*(2), 29–34.

Skinner, S. (1996). The world according to homeopathy. *Journal of Cardiovascular Nursing, 10*(3), 65–77.

Small, C.C. (1995). Appalachians. In J.N. Giger & R.E. Davidhizar (Eds.), *Transcultural nursing: Assessment and intervention* (pp. 263–280). St. Louis: Mosby.

Smit, H.F., Woerdenbag, H.J., Singh, R.H., Meulenbeld, G.J., Labadie, R.P., & Zwaving, J.H. (1995). Ayurvedic herbal drugs with possible cytostatic activity. *Journal of Enthopharmacology, 47*(2), 75–84.

Smith, L. (1997a). Critical thinking, health policy, and the Hmong culture group, part I. *Journal of Cultural Diversity, 4*(1), 5–12.

Smith, L. (1997b). Critical thinking, health policy, and the Hmong culture group, part II. *Journal of Cultural Diversity, 4*(2), 59–67.

Snow, L.F. (1983). Traditional health beliefs and practices among lower class Black Americans. *Western Journal of Medicine, 139,* 820–828.

Sobel, E., Huang, E.Y., & Wieting, C.B. (1997). Drop foot as a complication of acupuncture injury and intragluteal injection. *Journal of the American Podiatric Medical Association, 87*(2), 52–59.

Spanos, N.P., Burgess, C.A., & Burgess, M.F. (1994). Past-life identities, UFO abductions, and satanic ritual abuse: The social construction of memories. *International Journal of Clinical & Experimental Hypnosis, 42,* 433–446.

Stein, W. (1991). *Great mysteries. Shamans. Opposing viewpoints.* San Diego: Greenhaven Press.

Steiner, R. (1923). *How to know higher worlds: A modern path of initiation* (C. Bamford, Trans.). Hudson, NY: Anthroposophic Press.

Steiner, R.P. (1989). Tibetan medicine part IV: Pulse diagnosis in Tibetan medicine. *American Journal of Chinese Medicine, 17*(1–2), 79–84.

Stevenson, I. (1966). *Twenty cases suggestive of reincarnation.* New York: American Society for Psychical Research.

Stevenson, I. (1983). American children who claim to remember previous lives. *Journal of Nervous and Mental Disease, 171,* 742–748.

Stux, G., & Pomeranz, B. (1987). *Acupuncture: Textbook and atlas.* New York: Springer-Verlag, Inc.

Suarez, M., Raffaelli, M., & O'Leary, A. (1996). Use of folk healing practices by HIV-infected Hispanics living in the United States. *AIDS Care, 8,* 683–690.

Thomas, J. (1988). Kill or cure. *Nursing Times, 84*(7), 38–40.

Tokar, E. (1999). Seeing to the distant mountain: Diagnosis in Tibetan medicine. *Alternative Therapies in Health and Medicine, 5*(2), 50–58.

Tooker, E. (1979). *Native North American spirituality of the eastern woodlands. Sacred myths, dreams, visions, speeches, healing formulas, rituals, and ceremonies.* New York: Paulist Press.

Touchstone, S.J. (1983). *Herbal and folk medicine of Louisiana and adjacent states.* Princeton, LA: Folk-Life Books.

Tripp-Reimer, T. (1983). Retention of a folk-healing practice (matiasma) among four generations of urban Greek immigrants. *Nursing Research, 32*(2), 97–101.

Turner, R.N. (1990). *Naturopathic medicine: Treating the whole person.* Wellingborough, England: Thorsons Publishing.

Ulett, G.A., Han, J., & Han, S. (1998). Traditional and evidence-based acupuncture: History, mechanisms, and present status. *Southern Medical Journal, 91,* 1115–1120.

Ullman, D. (1991). *Discovering homeopathy: Medicine for the 21st century.* Berkeley, CA: North Atlantic Books.

Urba, S.G. (1996). Nonpharmacologic pain management in terminal care. *Clinics in Geriatric Medicine, 12,* 301–311.

U.S. Department of Commerce, Bureau of Census. (1993). *Population profiles of the United States: 1993.* Washington, DC: U.S. Government Printing Office.

U.S. Public Health Service. (1990). *Healthy people 2000: National health promotion and disease prevention objectives.* Washington, DC: U.S. Department of Health and Human Services.

Verma, V. (1995). *Ayurveda. A way of life.* York Beach, ME: Samuel Weiser, Inc.

Vilke, G.M., & Wulfert, E.A. (1997). Case reports of two patients with pneumothorax following acupuncture. *Journal of Emergency Medicine, 15,* 155–157.

Vincent, C., & Lewith, G. (1995). Placebo controls for acupuncture studies. *Journal of the Royal Society of Medicine, 88,* 603.

Vithoulkas, G. (1980). *The science of homeopathy.* New York: Grove.

Vogel, V.J. (1970). *American Indian medicine.* Norman, OK: University of Oklahoma Press.

Wallnöfer, H., & von Rottauscher, A. (1985). *Chinese folk medicine.* New York: Bell Publishing Co.

Walsh, R. (1996). Shamanism and healing. In B.W. Scotton, A.B. Chinen, & J.R. Battista (Eds.), *Textbook of transpersonal psychiatry and psychology* (pp. 96–103). New York: Basic Books, Inc.

Walsh, R.N. (1989). What is a shaman? Definition, origin, and distribution. *Journal of Transpersonal Psychology, 21*(1), 1–11.

Weisenthal, D.B. (1997, November-December). 5-day detox plan. *Natural Health,* pp. 86–91, 160–164.

Wendroff, A.P. (1997). Magico-religious mercury exposure. *Environmental Health Perspectives, 105,* 266.

Wenger, A.F.Z. (1995). Cultural context, health and health care decision making. *Journal of Transcultural Nursing, 7*(1), 3–14.

Werbach, M. (1993). *Nutritional influences on illness* (2nd ed.). Tarzana, CA: Third Line Press.

Westermeyer, J., & Her, C. (1996). English fluency and social adjustment among Hmong refugees in Minnesota. *Journal of Nervous and Mental Disease, 184*(2), 130–132.

Whitcomb, D.C., & Block, G.D. (1994). Association of acetaminophen hepatotoxicity with fasting and ethanol use. *JAMA, 272,* 1845–1850.

Wilbert, J. (1991). Does pharmacology corroborate the nicotine therapy and practices of South American shamanism? *Journal of Ethnopharmacology, 32,* 179–186.

Winkelman, M.J. (1990). Shamans and other "magico-religious" healers: A cross-cultural study of their origins, nature, and social transformations. *Ethos, 18,* 308–352.

Xu, R.S., Zhu, Q.Z., & Xie, Y.Y. (1985). Recent advances in studies on Chinese medicinal herbs with physiological activity. *Journal of Enthnopharmacology, 14*(2–3), 223–253.

Yoder, K.K. (1997). Nursing intervention considerations among Amish older persons. *Journal of Multicultural Nursing and Health, 3*(2), 48–52, 60.

Yu, C.M., Chan, J.C., & Sanderson, J.E. (1997). Chinese herbs and warfarin potentiation by "danshen." *Journal of Internal Medicine, 241,* 337–339.

Chapter Four

Manual Healing Methods

Georgia M. Decker, MS, RN, CS-ANP, AOCN

Introduction

Complementary and alternative therapies include many "hands-on" modalities, the origins of which date back thousands of years. These manual healing methods have been used to decrease stress, assist in relaxation, improve health, and prevent disease. The choice of method(s) should include an assessment of the patient's physical and emotional being, and patients should seek appropriately trained practitioners if considering any of these therapies.

Acupressure

The theory behind acupressure focuses on the belief that the body is a self-healing, dynamic whole composed of a network of interrelating energies. When this law of energies is evenly distributed, the body is able to maintain health.

Acupuncture and acupressure involve the same points on the body; the difference is that acupuncture uses special needles, while acupressure involves the firm pressure of the thumb and fingertips. Acupressure is the older of these two techniques and, although less commonly practiced, is considered to be effective in treating stress- and tension-related conditions (Jacobs, 1996).

Acupressure is similar to shiatsu in that it involves finger pressure on points throughout the body (Bradford, 1997; Rosenfeld, 1996). Unlike shiatsu, however, acupressure involves mostly the pressure from the thumb and fingertips. Acupressure also may incorporate massage along meridians (which are discussed in more detail in Chapter 3, "Alternative Systems of Medical Practice"). Some practitioners see acupressure as based in instinct—that is, the natural reaction to hold the body part that may be hurt or hurting. The Chinese have practiced self-acupressure for more than 5,000 years (Jacobs 1996).

According to the tenets of acupressure, tension is a stagnation of the body's flow, including meridians, nerves, blood, and lymphatic circulation. Stagnation can be caused by such factors as lack of exercise, poor diet, alcohol, and drugs (Jacobs, 1996). Psychological and emotional stress, including the stresses of everyday life, can cause blockage of the body's flow of impulses.

Acupressure points (also referred to as potent points) are places on the skin that are especially sensitive to, and therefore conduct, the body's bioelectrical impulses. The goal of acupressure is to stimulate these points with pressure to initiate the release of endorphins, which are neurochemicals that are thought to relieve the blockage. The sensation of pain is considered to be a symptom of blockage, and when interrupted, a simultaneous increase in the flow of blood and oxygen to the affected site occurs, which promotes healing. This has been referred to as "closing the gates" of the pain-signaling system (Jacobs, 1996).

Practitioners of acupressure believe that it has health-sustaining, illness-resisting benefits. It works by interrupting processes that inhibit the immune system. Body tension is believed to concentrate at acupressure points. As a point is pressed, the muscle releases, which causes the muscle fiber to lengthen and blood flow to increase. Toxins are released and then eliminated, and the flow of oxygen and nutrients to the site increases as a result (Jacobs, 1996).

Acupressure potent points can be used to manage stress, to relieve pain associated with injury, as adjunct therapy in chronic pain management, for the pain associated with arthritis and backache, and as a beauty treatment. Potent points affect a response in two ways. The "local point" is at the site of the pain or discomfort. The "trigger point" is at a site distant to the physical sensation that relieves discomfort through an electrical pathway called a meridian.

Anatomical landmarks are used to locate acupressure points. Points near a bone structure usually are found in an indentation, and those near a muscle are found in a muscle "knot," cord, or band (Jacobs, 1996). See Jacobs for some examples of potent point exercises.

Special Considerations

Many acupressure points are adjacent to others; therefore, it is possible to stimulate an undesired response. Choosing an appropriately prepared practitioner is essential.

Alexander Technique

Devised by an actor named Matthew Alexander at the turn of the century, this technique is a process of improving self-awareness of movement and its relationship to a person's health and performance. It is considered to be an educational process (as opposed to a therapy) that helps people to use their bodies more efficiently; it has been referred to as posture training, but this term is inaccurate. The primary principle of the Alexander Technique is that the mind and body form a complex and integrated whole. It is described in terms of the relationship between the head, neck, and back with the goal of directing the head away from the spine without tensing and narrowing the back. Usually, the balance of our head to our spine is innate. However, as we accommodate our posture to our environment, over time we lose this balance. The Alexander Technique does not claim to eliminate specific symptoms but rather to address the cause of an illness. According to Jacobs (1996), to fully understand this technique, one must experience it.

The goal of the Alexander Technique is to operationalize this neuromuscular/reorientation process. The central nervous system transmits and receives signals, and these signals are a form of thought. Learning will occur as the individual gains greater insight into habits that create unnecessary tension, physical or psychological distress, or pressure, pain, or "dis-ease" (i.e., with insight comes control) (Jacobs, 1996). Understanding the experience of clear thought and intention is a critical component of this learning: One can have a clear intention of not doing something as well as of doing something. Doing so sounds easier than it is because familiarity must be resisted when what is familiar is more stressful and less mechanically efficient. Continuous repetition of the less-stressful, more mechanically efficient action improves movement and attention while increasing awareness (Jacobs; Micozzi, 1996). Use of this technique requires time and discipline, and it is recommended to be used in activities of daily living. The Alexander Technique is interdisciplinary but is best known in the performing arts. Because the technique addresses key elements of human functioning, it has a wide variety of appropriate applications (Jacobs).

Special Considerations

The Alexander Technique should not be attempted without a teacher, who can provide essential feedback and oversee practice. A teacher can earn certification after a period of training that takes approximately three years. Although no standardized "prescription" exists, it is recommended that a student study for a minimum of six months (Jacobs, 1996). Lessons typically are delivered on a one-to-one basis. Teachers of the Alexander Technique use verbal and hands-on guidance to help students to develop new ways of moving. Gentle bodywork techniques such as the Alexander Technique have no defined contraindications, but individuals with chronic muscular pain or joint difficulties should consult with their healthcare providers prior to practicing such techniques (Cassileth, 1998). Such bodywork techniques may have significant implications for elderly individuals who experience problems with motor function.

Applied Kinesiology

Kinesiology is the study of movement. Physicians and physiotherapists have used some aspects of it to test range of motion and strength. It is a proven technique of muscle testing, training, and rehabilitation that is widely used for treating sports injuries (Rosenfeld, 1996). It is not used as a diagnostic tool for whole-body health and only claims to cure the particular muscle problem for which it is being used. Applied kinesiology is a diagnostic therapy that was first used in 1964 by George J. Goodheart, an American chiropractor, who believed that he could best assess a patient's health with muscle testing. A diagnostic therapy differs from a diagnostic tool in that a diagnostic therapy is used to analyze the cause of an illness to identify an imbalance before it becomes an illness rather than to diagnose a specific illness. Goodheart's colleagues disagreed, remaining strong in their belief that poor alignment of the spine was the basis of health problems. Goodheart developed a series of muscle tests that helped him to assess the health of the whole body. He believed that a central circulatory, lymphatic, endocrine, and nervous supply controlled by the same meridians used in acupressure connects muscles with internal organs; therefore, muscle function determines, and is indicative of, health (Rosenfeld).

Practitioners of applied kinesiology believe that they can diagnose various allergies, deficiencies, toxic states, and food sensitivities (Bradford, 1997; Rosenfeld, 1996). Diagnosis and treatment may vary from practitioner to practitioner. Testing is painless and involves the practitioner supporting the individual's limb to isolate the muscle to be tested. A point on the body that corresponds to that muscle and is linked by a meridian is then tapped while the practitioner simultaneously applies pressure to the limb. The individual is asked to resist the pressure; if he or she can resist, the body part is considered to be healthy. Inability to resist the pressure signifies an energy imbalance in the related body part (Bradford). For example, the strength of the deltoid muscle is believed to indicate lung function because the shoulder and the lung have common reflex stimulation. In another example, if an individual is sensitive to wheat and eats a piece of bread, the sensitivity would register in the intestines and then in the corresponding muscle in the legs.

Special Considerations

Applied kinesiology is not a "cure" for any illness. It focuses on finding and correcting subclinical conditions (e.g., food sensitivities, digestive problems, joint stiffness, headaches, phobias) before they evolve into illnesses. All weaknesses assessed by the tests are then addressed in order of priority. To provide sustained progress, the most important problems must be addressed first. All other problems are then addressed in descending order. Controversy exists regarding the effectiveness of applied kinesiology, but it is noninvasive and gentle and has no known side effects. There are no known contraindications. Do not confuse applied kinesiology with kinesiology. Kinesiology is a proven technique that is used by athletes and dancers (Rosenfeld, 1996).

Biodynamic Therapy

Biodynamic therapy employs special massage techniques and psychotherapy, the combination of which is believed to bring about emotional and physical healing. Biodynamic therapy was developed by Girda Boyisen, a Norwegian psychologist and physiotherapist who believed that emotional problems affect the muscles and organs of the body (Bradford, 1997). She saw the intestines as particularly vulnerable. She coined the term *biodynamics* to describe that energy flow connection of body, mind, and emotion. Biodynamic therapy combines massage and counseling to ease physical and emotional tension. The emotions, in fact, are central to this therapy. The biodynamic therapist believes that all emotion causes a physical reaction at the cellular level. As emotions resolve, the end products are eliminated through the intestines.

When one's life is burdened by stress, this "cleansing" malfunctions, and the body retains the end products. This retention has the potential to cause mental and physical problems. The initial visit to a biodynamic therapist includes an intestinal health history as well as past medical history (Jacobs, 1996). Through massage and counseling, this therapy promotes release of physical and emotional tension. Massage is believed to release the residue caught in body tissues.

Special Considerations

This therapy may be beneficial in relieving stress-related symptoms associated with lower-back pain, migraines, multiple sclerosis, and rheumatoid arthritis (Bradford, 1997). It is considered to be safe except for patients in advanced stages of disease. It is recommended for those with emotional or psychological problems that need to be resolved. Adequate and appropriate preparation of the practitioner is critical.

Chiropractic

Chiropractic is a therapy that focuses on the body's musculoskeletal system, primarily the spine and how it affects the nervous system. The term *chiropractic* comes from the Greek language and literally means "done by hands" (Bradford, 1997; Jacobs, 1996). Hippocrates, the father of modern medicine, practiced spinal manipulation; however, Daniel David Palmer is credited as being the father of chiropractic. Palmer was not a physician but rather a teacher with a keen interest in healing and bones and how bodies work, and he is said to have cured a janitor of deafness using spinal manipulation. The janitor had been deaf for 17 years and reported that his hearing loss had occurred after he felt something give or "pop" in his back. Palmer performed a vertebral adjustment on the man and, subsequently, the man's hearing returned. In curing the man's deafness, Palmer founded a completely new branch of medicine. He believed that improper alignment of the spine causes pressure on the nerves. This disrupts the normal flow of nerve impulses and interferes with normal function of muscles, respiration, heartbeat, digestion, arterial tone, and immunity. He believed that releasing the pressure on the nerves could restore health.

Chiropractic treatment is based upon the belief that the body's master system is the central nervous system (composed of the brain and spinal cord) and that all bodily functions are controlled and monitored under this master system. All illness is, then, a result of subluxation, a slippage of one of the 24 joints of the spinal cord. Generally, osteopaths and orthopedists do not endorse the concept of subluxation (Rosenfeld, 1996). They acknowledge that mechanical slippage of the spine can occur but do not consider it to be universal. Many allopathic physicians do not endorse chiropractic as an authentic treatment modality. However, chiropractors are eligible for state licensure, and an increasing number of insurers provide coverage for chiropractic therapy.

Chiropractic is complicated and highly specialized. It is similar to osteopathy but also differs in several key ways (see Figure 1). The chiropractor's goal is to restore the spine to normal as appropriate for an individual. Chiropractors use observation, palpation, and x-rays in their assessment. The three symptoms most frequently reported to chiropractors are pain, tightness or spasm, and weakness (Jacobs, 1996). The symptoms that most frequently are treated by chiropractors include arthritis, numbness/tingling, pain, sports injuries, strains, sprains, and stiffness. More than 100 chiropractic techniques exist; the most common can be classified as (a) direct thrust techniques, (b) indirect thrust techniques, or (c) soft tissue techniques (Bradford, 1997).

Figure 1. How Osteopathy Varies From Chiropractic	
Osteopathy	**Chiropractic**
Works on the entire body	Works primarily on the spine
Limits use of x-rays	Regularly uses x-rays
Relies on soft-tissue techniques	Relies on structural manipulation

Note. Based on information from Bradford, 1997.

Direct thrust techniques (also referred to as high-velocity thrusts) are rapid and forceful movements. The chiropractor will make contact using different parts of the hand on different joints. This movement may be accompanied by a loud cracking noise, which is believed to be the result of the bursting of gas bubbles in the spinal fluid. Indirect thrust techniques are used when direct thrust may be uncomfortable or not well-tolerated. In this method, the joint is gently stretched over a pad or towel; this process takes a few minutes to complete. Soft-tissue techniques usually are used prior to an adjustment to reduce spasm and aid in relaxing the joint but also are used to release trigger points (which are similar to acupuncture reflex points). Pain is reduced when the tension is eased. Current recognition of neurophysiology provides, at the very least, a theoretical basis for visceral organ response to adjustment.

Special Considerations

In 1994, a group of 21 physicians and 2 chiropractors developed guidelines for the Agency for Health Care Policy and Research, U.S. Department of Health and Human Services, on the treatment of acute lower-back pain; these guidelines included an endorsement of spinal manipulation (Micozzi, 1996). Central to chiropractic practice is the process of determining when spinal manipulation techniques are appropriate and which type of adjustment is indicated. The guidelines for chiropractic quality assurance and practice parameters identify situations in which high-velocity thrust adjustments are contraindicated (e.g., malignancies; bone or joint infections; acute myelopathy, bone diseases; acute cauda equina syndrome; acute fractures or dislocation; unstable healed fractures or dislocations; acute rheumatoid, rheumatoid-like, and other arthropathies; active juvenile vascular necrosis; unstable os odontoideum) (Micozzi). Low-force chiropractic adjustments are used when standard adjustments are contraindicated. Nonadjustive techniques also may be used under these circumstances.

Feldenkrais Method

The Feldenkrais Method is a training program that is designed to improve function, flexibility, coordination, and range of motion. No claims of medical therapy are made with this method. It is offered to both healthy and ill people of all ages. The most impressive results have been realized in people with neuromuscular disorders, such as multiple sclerosis and stroke. Many of its enthusiasts are elderly individuals who have gained improved movement and coordination through its use.

Moshe Feldenkrais was a Russian-born physicist who was left "crippled" after injuring his knees. He was determined to work again even though the medicine of his time was unable to restore full mobility. He began to study psychology, neurophysiology, physics, and biology and applied what he learned to body movement. He did succeed in walking again.

His method has two components: awareness through movement (ATM) and functional integration (FI). Participants usually start with ATM. In this component, the participant lies on his or her back and focuses on and feels the presence of various parts of the body. An instructor provides verbal cues as the participant repeats a sequence of simple movements. This component involves no hands-on experience with the instructor, whereas FI incorporates hands-on techniques. In FI, the participant lies, sits, or stands while the instructor verbally guides him or her through the same sequence of movements as in ATM, but the instructor also provides gentle manipulation of the participant's muscles and joints (Rosenfeld, 1996).

Special Considerations

Gentle bodywork techniques such as the Feldenkrais Method generally are considered to be safe. Improved movement in elderly participants has been reported (Rosenfeld, 1996). This is not a cure for any specific illness but has the potential to be helpful in treating motor problems. Patients should consult with their healthcare providers prior to practicing such techniques.

Massage Therapy

Massage is the specific manipulation of the body's soft tissues, using primarily the therapist's hands but sometimes the forearms, elbows, and feet, as well. Societal changes during the 1970s included an increased interest in physical fitness, personal improvement, improved health, and methods that complemented biomedicine; these changes contributed to an increased interest in massage. Massage provides the basis for shiatsu and other manual healing methods. Different types of massage exist, but each is grounded in the medium of touch (Jacobs, 1996). Massage consists of a series of techniques, but it involves not only mechanics; it also includes an artistic component. The touch used in massage involves applying varying degrees of pressure, which is determined by the sensitivity of the therapist to the client's needs. Sensitive touch allows the massage therapist to receive information about the body, such as the location of muscles or soft-tissue injury or other problems. Touch also is a form of communication. Massage can convey a positive emotional message: it communicates caring and can improve individuals' ability to cope with the isolation that some people feel. "Toxic touch" is the wrong kind of touch, is counterproductive, and may cause increased tension (Jacobs, 1996).

Massage therapy can be used in a variety of settings; desired outcomes range from reducing stress to healing sports injuries to treating specific problems. When performed on a regular basis, massage, combined with exercise and appropriate nutrition, can help to optimize and maintain health. Some of the benefits of massage include reduced muscle tension, edema, and stress; improved circulation, lymph movement, and mobility; enhanced digestion and intestinal function; and general relaxation (Jacobs, 1996). The client must communicate with the massage therapist (e.g., the degree of pressure used, any physical problems). Massage does not increase muscle strength, but it can promote recovery from the fatigue and minor aches and pains that can result from exercise. The relationship between the body's structure and function promotes the broad effects of this therapy. Massage is believed to counteract the effects of stress and increase relaxation, as well as to decrease the risk of stress-induced illness. Different types of touch are used in massage; Figure 2 summarizes the most common.

Figure 2. Basic Massage Techniques

Effleurage: Means light touch or stroke. There will be different pressure and speed of touch. Firm strokes improve circulation and stimulate lymphatic drainage. Slower strokes ease tension and reduce stress. Do not massage over varicose veins.

Petissage: Includes kneading and wringing. Both are techniques for deeper massage. It is most effective if preceded by effleurage. It releases tension from stiff muscles and improves circulation. Should not be used on recent injury, varicose veins, inflammation or scar tissue less than six months old. Avoid these techniques when massaging the abdomen.

Pressures: Involves applying a firm, penetrating amount of pressure to specific areas. The main types are: static and circular pressure. These techniques release muscular tension, loosen knots and increase blood flow to area. Do not use over bruised areas, where skin integrity is broken, on recent scars, or over varicose veins.

Percussion: Is a pounding stroke, used for stimulation. There are several types, and they are most effective when used on a large muscular area (e.g., buttocks). This method enhances circulation and improves tone. It should not be used on bony areas, bruised areas, or varicose veins.

Knuckling: Can be used with light or deep pressure. It is best used on the soles of the feet and palms of the hands. Some therapists use this method on the shoulders and chest, as well. It increases blood flow and decreases muscle tension. Do not use on abdomen, inflamed areas, broken skin, recent scars, or varicose veins.

Note. Based on information from Bradford, 1997.

More than 100 methods of massage exist; most can be categorized as traditional European, structural/functional, Oriental, or energetic. Many therapists, however, integrate a variety of methods in their work. Traditional European massage is based on conventional Western concepts of anatomy and physiology.

Swedish massage is the most common form of traditional European massage. This method uses long, gliding strokes, kneading, and friction, usually in the direction of blood flow toward the heart. It is very effective in promoting general relaxation and improving circulation and mobility (Jacobs, 1996). Swedish massage is vigorous and usually implemented as a full-body treatment.

Contemporary Western massage embraces the concepts of human functioning using a wide variety of techniques. Methods include, but are not limited to, neuromuscular massage, sports massage, deep-tissue massage, trigger-point massage, Esalen, and manual lymph drainage. Deep-tissue massage is indicated when the release of chronic patterns of muscular tension is desired. Sports massage uses techniques similar to Swedish and deep tissue that are adapted to address the needs of the athlete, but it also is beneficial for the effects suffered by the person who engages in periodic physical activity. Neuromuscular massage is a very specific form of deep-tissue massage that is used to decrease pain and may include trigger-point massage to release trigger points (knots of muscle tension). Manual lymph drainage is another very specific method of massage that employs light strokes. This method primarily is used for conditions associated with impaired lymphatic flow, such as lymphedema. Esalen massage focuses on creating deep relaxation and overall well-being. It is slow and rhythmic and focuses on the mind-body connection. Some therapists combine Esalen with Swedish massage. Chinese or Oriental massage (Thi Na, literally meaning "pushing and pulling") refers to a system of massage, manual acupuncture point stimulation, and manipulation. This method is a forceful, intense technique that most often is applied to limited areas of the body. Indications include orthopedic and neurological conditions; it also is used as an adjunct to acupuncture to improve mobility (Jacobs, 1996).

Massage therapists describe four stages of healing: (a) Relief—symptoms are eased, but the problem is still not solved; (b) Correction—of the underlying problem; (c) Strengthening—of the injured area to avoid reinjury; and (d) Maintenance—as the final stage of healing and the first step in prevention (Jacobs, 1996).

Massage can be a complement to any therapy by improving circulation and lymphatic drainage as well as reducing physiologic and psychological tension. Fugh-Berman (1997) suggested that the benefits of massage may be specific to those who receive them. Massage is not used to treat functional illnesses.

Special Considerations

Massage is considered to be safe for almost everyone when practiced by a qualified therapist. Qualified massage therapists can be located by contacting the American Massage Therapy Association (see contact information in the resource section at the end of this book). Massage therapists do not diagnose illness. Any injury resulting in the loss of function must be evaluated medically before using massage (Feltman, 1989). Massage should not be used for certain conditions/situations, including unhealed wounds, advanced osteoporosis, certain circulatory conditions, bleeding disorders, and when there is a possibility of the spread of disease via the circulatory or lymphatic system

Osteopathy

Doctors of Osteopathy (DO) account for approximately 5% of physicians in the United States; they have full legal and professional recognition, including unrestricted licenses (Micozzi, 1996). Osteopathy is patient-centered—not disease-centered—in its treatment. The originator, Andrew Taylor Still, was educated as an engineer prior to receiving formal medical training. After serving as an army surgeon and, later, seeing three of his children die, he became disillusioned with orthodox medicine and sought an alternative. Still's training as an engineer provided him with an understanding of body mechanics, and his belief in Hippocrates' claim that the "cause of disease lives within the body" convinced him that the answers he sought could be found within the human body (Bradford, 1997). He believed that structure governed function, and this belief is one of the basic principles of contemporary osteopathy. Still considered the spine to be the most important of the body's bony structures because the spine protects the spinal cord, and the spinal cord connects the brain with the central nervous system. He called his techniques and beliefs *osteopath,* which literally means "bone disease" (Bradford; Jacobs, 1996). In 1874, Still began practicing a system emphasizing health rather than disease and developed a way to improve the body's own self-healing mechanisms, which involved palpation of the musculoskeletal system to identify dysfunction and then manipulation to reestablish optimal function.

Osteopathy is a healing system that stresses the importance of the neuromuscular system in diagnosis and treatment. Osteopathic principles and practices and osteopathic manipulation treatment (OMT) are integral components of DO training (Jacobs, 1996). According to Jacobs, the tenets of osteopathic medicine are

1. The body is an integrated unit.
2. Structure and function are interrelated.
3. The body has self-healing, self-regulating mechanisms.

DOs use traditional treatment modalities, but the components of the treatment plan are individualized in keeping with the osteopathic philosophy. The osteopathic physician does not address one organ system or structure to the exclusion of another but rather views the body as an integral unit. OMT may or may not be a component of osteopathic treatment (Jacobs).

Osteopathy uses a series of established manipulative techniques. Light or heavy pressure may be used. Somatic dysfunction is the osteopathic "lesion," and the diagnosis is based upon the identification of asymmetry, restricted movement, and textural changes. Soft-tissue manipulation is similar to massage but only is applied to areas that need it with a specific response as the goal of therapy. Manipulative therapy is useful for maintaining function and correcting dysfunction (Bradford, 1997). Neuromuscular techniques involve the DO using his or her thumb to probe tissue for stress or tension. Articulatory techniques are gentle and rhythmic. Ligaments tend to resist short, quick movements, but this technique allows for gradual restoration of function. The high-velocity thrust is a technique that is seen in chiropractic as well as osteopathy and primarily is used on the spine. A cracking or popping sound characteristically accompanies this movement. Indirect techniques are so subtle that patients may fall asleep during treatment. Not all osteopaths use these techniques; indications for use include treatment of muscles or loose connective tissue. All OMTs are based on a complete structural assessment that may include radiographic or magnetic imaging as well as laboratory studies (Bradford).

Osteopathic medicine is centered on holism, health versus disease, and homeostasis. Osteopathy is believed to provide relief for symptoms of muscular pain, joint pain, backache, neck problems, sciatica, sports injuries, vertigo, migraines, premenstrual syndrome, digestion problems (including constipation), thoracic outlet syndrome, and respiratory and cardiac conditions, among others (Bradford, 1997; Jacobs, 1996). Osteopathic technique can be adapted to treat anyone, but all treatment, to be safe, must be provided by a DO.

Cranial osteopathy is a subtle form of OMT that was developed by William Garner Sutherland, a disciple of Andrew Still. It is a specialized technique used to manipulate the bones of the skull with an extremely light touch (Bradford, 1997); in fact, people often report that they can barely feel it. Critics question whether a touch so light as to be barely perceptible can produce therapeutic benefit. Craniosacral therapy evolved from cranial osteopathy. An osteopath may use cranial techniques; however, a craniosacral therapist may or may not have a background in osteopathy. Therefore, practitioner education and training can be notably different (Bradford).

By experimenting on himself, Sutherland discovered that compressing the skull could have a profound mental and physical impact. He then found that cerebrospinal fluid had rhythms, which he named "the breath of life" because they appeared to be influenced by breathing; he described this impulse as cranial rhythmic impulse (Bradford, 1997). Using gentle manipulation of the skull, he was able to alter the rhythm of the flow of fluid, which he thought might stimulate the body's ability to self-heal.

Cranial techniques are used to relieve symptoms of biomechanical imbalance and nerve dysfunction, including pain, numbness, and weakness. They are believed to reduce edema, improve cognition, and enhance breathing and energy levels. This modality stimulates the body's ability to heal and can be used to treat tinnitus, vertigo, colitis, urinary incontinence, and painful masses. It also can be useful as a treatment for pain conditions, including lower-back pain, neck pain, migraines, TMJ dysfunction, and other facial pain (Bradford).

Special Considerations

Identification of an appropriately trained and licensed practitioner is essential for safe, successful treatment.

Reflexology and Zone Therapy

Reflexology has its roots in the ancient civilizations of Egypt, China, and India, as well as in Native American culture. However, it essentially had no impact in the West until the early 20th century, when William Fitzgerald, an ear, nose, and throat specialist, became interested in zone therapy (Jacobs, 1996; Rosenfeld, 1996). Zone therapy provides the foundation for reflexology. In zone therapy, the entire body is divided into 10 vertical zones. Fitzgerald discovered that by putting pressure on one part of the body, it was possible to relieve pain in other parts of the body in the same zone.

Contemporary reflexology is the practice of applying specific pressure to points on the feet and hands—usually feet (see Figure 3). It is a holistic modality, for it addresses the needs of the entire body. To understand reflexology, one must picture the human body superimposed on the feet. The practitioner correlates sensitive areas of the feet with body parts (see Figure 4). The pressure may vary from heavy to light, depending on the reflexologist. The original concept involved heavy pressure at the tender spots; more recently, however, lighter pressure is applied to avoid creating an additional stressor—pain. Reflexologists do not diagnose, prescribe, or cure. An appropriately trained reflexologist does have an understanding of the relationship between structure and function. Reflexology is more than a foot massage with pressure applied to tender areas. Practitioners see the foot as a guide, and a session involves an "assessment" of the entire foot. Exactly how reflexology works is unclear, but it is believed to help to restore balance in the body by restoring energy flow and enhancing health. It also may enhance blood and lymphatic flow. Skeptics believe that reflexology "works" because caring touch is involved, and touch has been proven to be therapeutic (Rosenfeld, 1996). This therapy does involve relaxation techniques, which can be very effective. Reflexology techniques can be performed on oneself, but another person can perform these techniques more easily.

Reflexology can be used to ease symptoms of many conditions, including digestive disorders, such as diarrhea and constipation; stress-related disorders, such

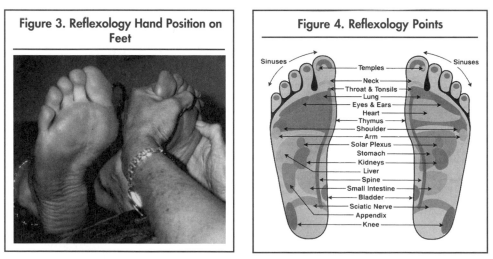

Figure 3. Reflexology Hand Position on Feet

Figure 4. Reflexology Points

as migraines and asthma; chronic pain; allergy; skin conditions, including psoriasis; menstrual irregularities, and fatigue (Jacobs, 1996; Rosenfeld, 1996).

Special Considerations

Reflexology is not intended as a cure but rather to provide symptomatic relief. Patients who are pregnant, have had recent foot injury, are ill with a fever, or have gallstones or kidney stones should not undergo reflexology until the condition is no longer present. Reflexology is not recommended for those who have had recent surgery until the incision is fully healed. Patients with phlebitis or deep vein thrombosis should avoid this therapy. Reflexologists come from a variety of backgrounds. Unless using this therapy for general relaxation, an individual should be sure that the practitioner is properly trained and has an understanding of the relationship between the body's structure and function.

Metamorphic Technique

Metamorphic technique also focuses on the feet as reflective of the whole person. Unlike the reflexologist, the practitioner of metamorphic technique does not concentrate on painful areas of the feet; rather, the technique simply acknowledges that they exist. Practitioners prefer the title "catalyst" rather than "therapist" because they do not see their role as identifying what needs to be healed but rather stimulating the person's own healing capacity. The main reflexes used are those along the spinal cord.

Special Considerations

Metamorphic technique is not a cure but rather an aid in coping with chronic conditions. As with all manual healing methods, the preparation and training of the practitioner are central to safe, effective results.

Rolfing (Structural Integration)

This method was developed by Ida Rolf in the United States in the 1930s. Rolf discovered that if the connective tissue (fascia) around the binding of each muscle was manipulated, then the body could be realigned. She recognized that when people are well-aligned, they move in harmony with gravity. Recognition of gravity's impact on body structure distinguishes Rolfing from other types of manual healing methods (Bradford, 1997). The fascia is loose and mobile, which allows free movement of muscles and joints. Chronic stress or inactivity can cause fascia to thicken and form adhesions; that is, layers stick to each other and form what is felt as a "knot" in a muscle (Jacobs, 1996). In Rolfing, a body that can spontaneously heal itself is one that functions well, with the force of gravity flowing evenly throughout. Rolfing is considered to be a philosophical position as much as a hands-on therapy (Jacobs).

The goal of this therapy is to reverse unhealthy misalignment by manipulating the connective tissue, thereby allowing the body to move more appropriately and to restore a state of balance. Rolfing is not aimed at specific conditions or diagnoses but rather at the restoration of the state of structural balance. Individuals undergoing this therapy have reported relief from back, neck, shoulder, and joint pain (Jacobs, 1996). Practitioners believe that any condition involving or resulting from poor posture will benefit from Rolfing. A common misconception regarding Rolfing is that it consists of painful pressure applied to the client. In truth, the Rolfer's visual assessment is the primary tool, and it is a "refined" pressure that is applied to soften and lengthen fascia.

Special Considerations

Rolfing is considered to be safe for adults and children, except for patients who have organic or inflammatory conditions, such as cancer and rheumatoid arthritis. Recent research conducted at the University of Maryland revealed that the changes made by Rolfing are long-lasting and may not require maintenance sessions (Jacobs, 1996). An appropriate practitioner is central to safe treatment (see the resource list at the end of this book).

Trager Method (Psychophysical Integration)

This method was developed by Milton Trager, an MD who also embraced the teachings of Ayurvedic medicine. This technique involves the Trager practitioner working in a meditative state. The client's body is gently and rhythmically rocked, bounced, and shaken to ease movement, loosen joints, increase range of motion, and decrease tension (Jacobs, 1996; Rosenfeld, 1996). After the hands-on portion of the session, the client is provided with instruction on "Mentastics," a form of mental gymnastics and self-directed movement that Trager believed would reinforce the hands-on portion of the session. He also believed that Mentastics could slow the aging process (Jacobs; Rosenfeld).

Tragerwork is believed to help people with asthma, autism, muscular dystrophy, multiple sclerosis, and other neuromuscular disorders by loosening joints, releasing tension, and improving range of motion. Most of this is documented as anecdotal case histories (Rosenfeld, 1996).

Special Considerations

Special considerations are similar to those of other bodywork. Tragerwork has the potential to improve muscle function and reduce the symptoms of neuromuscular diseases, but it is not a cure for any disease or condition. Rosenfeld (1996) suggested that it be considered as an extension of physiotherapy.

Therapeutic Touch

Therapeutic touch was derived from the ancient practice of laying on of hands. The fundamental assumption is that a universal life energy sustains all life. In 1975, Delores Krieger, a professor of nursing, and Dora Kunz, a clairvoyant, hypothesized that the ability to assist with healing is innate in us all and, subsequently, founded therapeutic touch (Kreiger, 1979). The *American Journal of Nursing* published an article by Krieger (1975) that described a significantly greater increase in the hemoglobin levels of patients who received therapeutic touch as compared to those who received routine nursing care. Although it was considered unorthodox at the time, therapeutic touch since has been integrated into the healthcare system.

Within the context of therapeutic touch, healing is described as restoration of balanced energy flow achieved through interrelated, simultaneous processes that (a) assess the person's energies or presence of congestion or deficit, (b) clear congestion, (c) transfer life energy into depleted areas, and (d) balance the energy flow (Macrae, 1993). The therapeutic touch practitioner must be in a calm, focused state to begin. The hands are held three to five inches above the body, and the entire body must be assessed even when a patient has a specific symptom. In a healthy person, the energy flow "feels" balanced, whereas in an ill individual, the practitioner realizes different sensations that indicate difficulties with energy flow. When the practitioner passes his or her hands through a person's energy field, he or she may feel heaviness, pressure, or heat in certain areas. Gentle, downward motions of the hands clear this because energy congestion tends to travel from the head to the toes (Macrae; Kreiger, 1975, 1979). Before the assessment is initiated, the therapeutic touch practitioner should establish his or her intent to be an energy conductor. Practitioners believe that as soon as a person who has a desire to help moves toward the patient, the patient may start to draw energy. Compassion opens people to one another.

Special Considerations

A therapeutic touch treatment may need to be interrupted prior to completion and may conclude if the session becomes too intense for the individual (Macrae,

1993). Therapeutic touch has been shown to be effective in the treatment of pain, anxiety, headaches, insomnia, and hypertension, as well as in healing wounds, increasing hemoglobin count, promoting relaxation, and easing loneliness in the elderly (Macrae). It is considered to be complementary in the care of upper respiratory illnesses, allergy, musculoskeletal conditions, labor and delivery, nausea, fever, and premenstrual syndrome. In situations involving the frail, the elderly, babies, or individuals with psychosis, shock, or head injuries, this therapy only should be used with extreme sensitivity on the part of the practitioner (Kreiger, 1979; Macrae).

Reiki

Reiki means "universal life energy." Derived from Japanese, it is an ancient healing art in which the healer is thought to manipulate energy. The energy—not the healer—actually affects healing. The purpose of Reiki is to relieve the body of physical, emotional, and spiritual "blockages." The healing of illness takes place by working on the emotional, mental, and spiritual levels rather than only on the physical. Reiki uses five premises or assumptions (Finley, 1992):

1. There is an energy of many unique properties, some of which are applicable to both medical and psychological conditions.
2. This energy has a source.
3. This source can be contacted and tapped.
4. A person easily can be taught to utilize this energy.
5. The effects of applying this energy are palpable, although subjective.

One major difference between Reiki and many other healing systems is that Reiki energy comes *through* rather than *from* the practitioner; this is called "channeling." If one is not generating the energy, one is less likely to be drained, or harmed, by channeling it. This unique feature allows practitioners to use Reiki on themselves or to help others without concern for their own personal energy. Reiki principles also state that the universal energy is not filtered through the user's conscious or unconscious belief systems. The energy is then said to remain pure and can find its way wherever and however it is needed without regard to the practitioner's or client's faith or religion.

Reiki is reported as being used to treat a wide variety of medical conditions and, according to Finley (1992), is particularly helpful for reducing pain and stress, increasing vitality, and bolstering the client's outlook. The Reiki session consists of the practitioner gently placing his or her hands on the client in a series of 12 positions. Five minutes are spent on each (time and positions may be varied for special needs). The client remains fully clothed at all times; no pressure is applied to the body, nor is there any manipulation or massage. The treatment is performed on a standard massage table, and the environment is kept as quiet and soothing as possible. After a session, the client should feel relaxed and peaceful.

Special Considerations

Because this therapy involves no physical manipulation, Reiki has the potential for use in situations in which traditional massage is not recommended or tolerated.

Summary

Manual healing methods appeal to us because our strongest instinct as human beings is to touch and be touched. The therapeutic value of some of these therapies is scientifically proven, while others are yet to be proven. The use of a particular manual therapy for a specific illness has been proven in some cases.

Research is being conducted, and the body of knowledge will increase as the outcomes become verified. As with all complementary/alternative therapies, we must assume responsibility for verifying the credentials and training of the practitioner.

References

Bradford, M. (Ed.). (1997). *Alternative health care.* San Diego: Thunderbay Press.

Cassileth, B.R. (1998). *The alternative medicine handbook: The complete reference guide to alternative and complementary therapies.* New York: Norton.

Feltman, J. (Ed.). (1989). *Hands-on healing: Massage remedies for hundreds of health problems.* Emmaus, PA: Rodale Press.

Finley, S. (1992, March/April). Secrets of Reiki. *Health and Healing.*

Fugh-Berman, A. (1997). *Alternative medicine: What works.* Baltimore: Williams &Wilkins.

Gordon, J.S. (1996). *Manifesto for a new medicine: Your guide to healing partnerships and the use of alternative therapies.* Reading, MA: Addison-Wesley.

Jacobs, J. (Ed.). (1996). *The encyclopedia of alternative medicine: A complete family guide to complementary therapies.* Boston: Carlton Books Ltd.

Krieger, D. (1975). Therapeutic touch: The imprimatur of nursing. *American Journal of Nursing, 75,* 784–787.

Kreiger, D. (1979). *The therapeutic touch. How to use your hands to help or heal.* Englewood Cliffs, NJ: Prentice Hall.

Macrae, J. (1993). *Therapeutic touch: A practical guide.* New York: Knopf.

Micozzi, M. (Ed.). (1996). *Fundamentals of complementary and alternative medicine.* New York: Simon & Schuster

Rosenfeld, I. (1996). *Dr. Rosenfeld's guide to alternative medicine.* New York: Random House.

Chapter Five

Pharmacologic and Biologic Therapies

Wende L. Levy, RN, MS, and
Georgia M. Decker, MS, RN,
CS-ANP, AOCN

Introduction

Rosenfeld (1996) referred to "the lure of the cure," and pharmacologic and biologic therapies represent much of the lure-and-cure phenomenon. The claims to cure everything from obesity to cancer provide the hope that many seek. It has long been recognized that people with debilitating or terminal illnesses are easy targets for these therapies. On the other side of this argument is the adage that the "truth must go through three stages: first, it is rejected; second, it is violently opposed; and third, it is accepted as self-evident" (Quillin & Quillin, 1994, p xii). Many pharmacologic and biologic therapies are in stages one and two. This is because generally there is a lack of scientific research to substantiate the claims made by these therapies. This chapter addresses some of the most controversial of these therapies.

Oxidation

Oxidation is a process that is essential to life as we know it. Deep breathing exercises are prescribed for patients who are recovering from surgery and with certain respiratory conditions. Altman (1995) reported that many diseases result from anaerobic pathogens and oxygen deficiencies. German biochemist Otto Warburg identified that oxygen deficiency and cell death were integral components of the cancer process. He demonstrated that cancer cells cannot survive in an oxygen-rich environment (Diamond, Cowden, & Goldberg, 1997). Bio-oxidative therapies are believed to increase oxygen metabolism and stimulate oxygen release into the blood and cells of the human body. This is believed to decrease the ability of pathogens to survive in an oxygen-rich environment, resulting in an overall increase in the immunologic response (Diamond et al.).

Two of the oxidative therapies most often used in complementary and alternative therapies are ozone and hydrogen peroxide.

Ozone

Ozone (chemical name: O_3), a highly active form of oxygen, is a pale-blue gas that becomes liquid at low temperatures. It provides the protective layer around the earth's upper atmosphere by absorbing ultraviolet radiation. Atmospheric ozone combines with vehicular exhaust, creating photochemical smog. Many scientific studies have focused on the negative effects of ozone; however, it has some potentially useful medical effects that must be acknowledged.

Ozone in Medicine

Ozone first was used as a disinfectant in operating rooms in 1956, and by 1960 it was used for water purification because of its antiviral, antibacterial, and antifungal properties. Studies began as early as 1915 to identify uses for ozone in medicine. Mucous colitis and fistulae were treated with ozone by rectal insufflation in 1932 (Altman, 1995).

Most research on ozone has been conducted in Europe. Ozone is believed to provide elements that improve circulation, stimulate cellular oxygen exchange and oxygen balance, and regulate immune function (Altman, 1995). Fritz Kramer, a German dentist, reported using ozone for wound cleansing and to improve healing. Methods of delivery of ozone include as a mouth rinse, as a spray for disinfection, via intramuscular injections, and by rectal insufflation (Altman).

Rectal insufflation is considered to be the safest method of delivery. In this method, ozone and oxygen are administered by way of a rectal tube through the rectum and absorbed by the body through the intestines. Disorders such as ulcerative colitis are treated with 100–800 ml of oxygen and ozone administered over two minutes by rectal insufflation and retained in the intestines for 10–20 minutes (Altman, 1995).

Intramuscular ozone and oxygen have been used to treat allergic and inflammatory conditions (Altman, 1995). Willner (1994) suggested that low doses of ozone stimulate the immune system, while large doses inhibit the immune system. In Europe, ozone also has been used to treat some cancers. The theory, as Willner reported, is that ozone provides the cancer cell with "toxic waste" while providing normal cells with the oxygen essential for life.

Cellular Oxygen Deficiency and Cancer

Otto Warburg, in 1931, identified that oxygen deficiency and cell fermentation, which occur when supplies of oxygen at the cellular level are diminished, are agents in the cancer process (Diamond et al., 1997). He believed that normal cells require oxygen but that cancer cells can live without oxygen. When the body is out of balance, it uses oxygen less effectively. Cells that are deprived of oxygen use sugar fermentation to provide energy. Cancer cells then produce lactic acid as a by-product of the fermentation process and can contain up to 10 times the amount of lactic acid as normal, healthy tissues (Diamond et al.). This results in a decrease in the body's ability to maintain an acid-base balance. Several environmentalists have theorized that the decrease in oxygen levels and the increase in carbon dioxide levels in the atmosphere is one of the reasons for the increase in the incidence of cancers.

Humans experience oxygen deficiency through long-term exposure to air pollution from automobiles, factory emissions, and tobacco smoke. The oxygen-rich environment of foods also is altered by cooking, processing, or preserving. Additionally, a sedentary lifestyle and shallow breathing can contribute to a decreased oxygen supply.

A method of administering ozone therapy is to bubble ozone gas through water. The water is then used to cleanse wounds and burns and to expedite healing in slow-healing wounds (Altman, 1995). Skin conditions can be treated with oil that has had ozone added to it.

Hydrogen Peroxide

Hydrogen peroxide (chemical name: H_2O_2) easily mixes in water and is clear and colorless. When ozone is bubbled through cold water, it creates hydrogen peroxide. Thus, hydrogen peroxide's ability to oxidize is similar to ozone's. It reacts with other substances easily and is viricidal, bactericidal, and fungicidal; it also has the potential to be cytotoxic to cancer cells (Altman, 1995).

Hydrogen peroxide is a natural product of the earth's environment. It is a component of plant life and is found in vegetables and fruits (Altman, 1995). Hydrogen peroxide stimulates oxidative enzymes, aids in cell transport, acts as a hormonal messenger, regulates heat production, stimulates and regulates energy production, and has many important metabolic functions (Altman). Granulocytes produce hydrogen peroxide as a product of cellular metabolism, as a regulator of hormonal levels, and in the regulation of blood sugar and energy production. Hydrogen peroxide can be administered intravenously, orally, topically, and by direct injection into a joint.

Hydrogen Peroxide in Medicine

Hydrogen peroxide is used in various concentrations for different purposes. Three-percent hydrogen peroxide is a diluted form that is sold commercially and used to cleanse wounds. The bubbling action of the solution is the release of the oxygen. The 6% solution is used as a bleaching agent, primarily in the cosmetic industry. Higher grades of hydrogen peroxide are considered chemical agents and must be used according to directions. Rocket fuel, for example, is made from 90% hydrogen peroxide.

The British physician T.H. Oliver was the first to use hydrogen peroxide for medical purposes (to treat pneumonia) in 1920 (Altman, 1995). Hydrogen peroxide was used in the United States in 1920 to treat cancer (Diamond et al., 1997); however, the medical community did not embrace early studies. In the 1960s, studies in the use of hydrogen peroxide conducted at Baylor University demonstrated that cells containing higher levels of oxygen were more susceptible to radiation, resulting in more favorable therapeutic results. In subsequent studies, the same physicians found that IV administration of hydrogen peroxide could achieve the same effect at a lower cost. Additional studies by researchers at Baylor concluded that IV administration of hydrogen peroxide also could be beneficial to patients who had had a cardiac event (Altman). Administration of hydrogen peroxide had an energizing effect on the heart muscle, thereby reducing myocardial ischemia. The treatment of atherosclerosis with hydrogen peroxide also was studied at Baylor. Researchers found a long-term decrease in plaque buildup with hydrogen peroxide use. These results were considered significant by the researchers but were not embraced by mainstream medicine (Diamond et al.).

Being both an oxygenator and oxidizer, hydrogen peroxide has been used to treat many diseases. The public is ill-informed about the benefits and treatment effects of 30% reagent grade or 35% food-grade hydrogen peroxide. Through their bio-oxidative effects, these grades of hydrogen peroxide kill fungi, bacteria, parasites, viruses, and certain cancer cells. Some researchers postulate that hydrogen peroxide therapy has implications in the treatment of certain viral conditions, allergies, Alzheimer's disease, angina, asthma, cardiac conditions, cerebral vascular disease, chronic obstructive pulmonary disease, recurrent Epstein Barr infection, chronic pain, cluster and migraine headaches, diabetes mellitus, emphysema, herpes simplex and zoster, influenza, Parkinson's disease, peripheral vascular disease, and rheumatoid arthritis (Altman, 1995).

IV Hydrogen Peroxide

When given intravenously, 30% hydrogen peroxide is diluted and made into a stock solution (see Figure 1). This solution is sterilized by passing it through a micropore filter to remove any particulate matter and then refrigerated. The strength of the final solution administered to patients is 0.03% and is obtained by mixing the stock solution with 5% dextrose in water or normal saline. The length and number of times of administration varies depending on the condition being treated. IV administration of hydrogen peroxide is considered to be the most effective route (Altman, 1995).

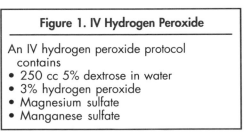

Figure 1. IV Hydrogen Peroxide

An IV hydrogen peroxide protocol contains
- 250 cc 5% dextrose in water
- 3% hydrogen peroxide
- Magnesium sulfate
- Manganese sulfate

Oral Hydrogen Peroxide

Many dental advocates tout hydrogen peroxide as a mouthwash and an ingredient in toothpaste. Oral ingestion, however, remains a subject of great controversy (Douglass, 1996). Hydrogen peroxide is measured by the drop for oral administration and should be mixed in distilled water. Advocates of oral administration caution against mixing it with juice or milk or using flavoring because this will create oxidation and destroy the benefit of administration. Also, hydrogen peroxide should not be administered in water containing iron because free radicals will be produced. Free radicals have been shown to increase the risk of some cancers and other disease processes (Altman, 1995).

Photooxidation

Also known as ultraviolet blood irradiation, photooxidation is based upon the knowledge that ultraviolet light can kill most bacteria. The patient's blood (100–200 cc) is drawn into a sterile syringe or container after the patient receives an ozone or hydrogen peroxide infusion. It is then run through special equipment that exposes the blood to ultraviolet light. The blood then is reinjected into the patient. This is a closed system to avoid the risk of contamination (Bock & Sabvin, 1997).

Special Considerations

Ozone is toxic if inhaled. IV hydrogen peroxide may cause venous irritation. The safety of any oxidative therapy is directly related to the practitioner's expertise.

Cell Treatment

Cell treatment was developed in the1930s by Paul Niehan (Heimlich, 1990). This therapy involves the administration of animal fetal cells by intramuscular injection. The cells migrate by genetic coding (biochemical, physiological, and bioelectrical properties). These tissues are able to integrate with corresponding tissues (Willner, 1994). Figure 2 describes the process and patient instructions.

Figure 2. Patient Teaching for Cell Therapy

Prior to therapy:
A history and physical examination will be completed.
Laboratory tests will be conducted.
• Complete blood count
• Sedimentation rate
• Chem screen
• Urinalysis
Cells to be used will be identified.

Patient instructions:
Take 10 grams of vitamin C daily in divided doses for five days prior to therapy and 10 days following therapy.
Avoid the use of tobacco, alcohol, antibiotics, and hot baths and avoid sun exposure for at least 10 days after therapy.
While reactions are rare and usually mild, they may include fever, localized swelling, redness, itching, and soreness.
Cells are injected with a local anesthetic for comfort.
Maintain complete bed rest for two days (bathroom privileges are permitted).
Rest on the third day.

Note. From *The Cancer Solution* (pp. 47–48), by R. Willner, 1994, Boca Raton, FL: Peltec Publishing Co., Inc. Copyright 1994 by Peltec Publishing Co., Inc. Adapted with permission.

Special Considerations

There is a risk of infection from contaminated specimens. Special considerations are the same as for any intramuscular injection.

Chelation Therapy

Chelation therapy uses a synthetic amino acid (ethylene diamine tetra-acetic acid [EDTA]) to remove toxic metals from the body (see Figure 3). It was approved in 1950 by the U.S. Food and Drug Administration (FDA) for treatment of heavy metal toxicity. Other uses for chelation therapy accidentally were discovered after patients who were treated with this therapy for lead poisoning noted improvements in their vision,

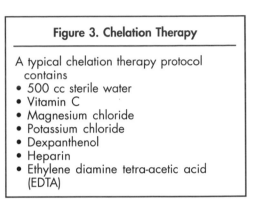

Figure 3. Chelation Therapy

A typical chelation therapy protocol contains
- 500 cc sterile water
- Vitamin C
- Magnesium chloride
- Potassium chloride
- Dexpanthenol
- Heparin
- Ethylene diamine tetra-acetic acid (EDTA)

ability to distinguish smells, memory, and ability to problem-solve. Also noted was an increased ability to perform activities that previously had caused the pain associated with angina and intermittent claudication. These results intrigued cardiologists, who then began to explore the potential benefits of this therapy for treating circulatory conditions. While use of chelation therapy for lead poisoning is an accepted medical practice, other uses of chelation therapy are more controversial and are not FDA-approved at this time. In coronary artery disease and other circulatory diseases, chelation is believed to restore circulation by dissolving the plaque that has formed in the walls of the arteries.

Albert Boyle and Gordon B. Myers were two of the first cardiologists to consider and investigate the benefits of chelation therapy as a method for treating circulatory problems (Brecher & Brecher, 1997; Cranton, 1997). Research showed that patients demonstrated signs of increased blood flow to extremities following chelation therapy, resulting in a decrease in pain with exercise (intermittent claudication) and improved temperature to the extremities. Also noted were an increased exercise tolerance and the ability to exercise without the presence of angina or shortness of breath. Two researchers, H. Richard Casdorph and E.W. McDonagh, were able to demonstrate the positive effects of this therapy on blood flow (Cranton). Using radioactive isotopes, Casdorph demonstrated increased blood flow to the heart by measuring the ejection fraction both pre- and post-treatment. This study confirmed the results that had been demonstrated when chelation was used to treat lead poisoning. Chelation therapy improves blood cholesterol ratios and lowers lipids and triglycerides. Chelation has been shown to increase blood flow through the body and is used in the treatment of Parkinson's disease, diabetes, multiple sclerosis, and arthritis (Cranton).

One obstacle to using chelation therapy is the cost. Most forms of insurance, including Medicare, do not cover this treatment. The insurance industry has declared that it is not medically indicated or necessary. Medicare may cover chelation for specific emergency conditions and only if administered for emergency treatment of hypercalcemia, control of ventricular arrhythmias, and heart block related to digitalis toxicity or heavy metal toxicity (Cranton, 1997). Chelation has not met the standards as reported by government scientists to receive approval for the treatment of atherosclerosis. Another risk is that chelation therapy can be nephrotoxic; close monitoring of renal function during therapy is imperative.

To be evaluated as a potential candidate for chelation therapy, the patient must complete a detailed medical history, including a family and lifestyle assessment. A complete physical assessment is performed, including peripheral vascular testing and an electrocardiogram. A chest x-ray and cardiac stress test also may be completed. Adequate renal function must be confirmed. Once the practitioner reviews the results, a schedule of treatments is prescribed. The number of treatments is individualized, but approximately 30 treatments typically are given over three to five months (Brecher & Brecher, 1997; Cranton, 1997).

During the chelation infusion, the patient will sit in a reclining chair while an IV is started. The infusion rate for the therapy is slow (approximately one drop per second). The infusion will contain EDTA and various amounts of vitamins and minerals (Cranton, 1997). Patients are asked to drink water and snack continuously during the infusion and to eat a meal prior to the infusion. The increase in fluid intake is to support renal function. Eating during therapy helps to prevent possible hypoglycemia. Each treatment takes approximately three hours.

The benefits from each infusion are directly proportional to the cumulative number of infusions. A break in therapy can be taken, but patients using chelation therapy to treat a specific disease are encouraged to maintain the treatment schedule for maximum effect. Patients who use chelation therapy for prevention of disease require fewer treatments with longer time intervals between infusions. All individuals who are receiving chelation should be closely followed by their healthcare team and should immediately report any change in medications or symptoms to their healthcare provider.

Chelation therapy is thought by some to be a means for eliminating the need for bypass surgery for coronary artery disease (Cranton, 1997). At this time, chelation is used more as a means to forestall or supplement surgical intervention than to totally eliminate the need for bypass surgery. Chelation therapy can be used as a holistic approach to cardiac disease and has been used by patients when surgery is deemed too risky.

Special Considerations

Chelation therapy should be prescribed and administered only by a certified practitioner (certification is through the American College for Advancement in Medicine). The chelation formula is individualized based upon history, physical, and laboratory data, and kidney function must be closely monitored.

Antineoplastons

In the 1960s, Stanislaw Burzynski first isolated several peptides—chains of amino acids that are considered the building blocks of protein—from urine (Diamond et al., 1997). These peptides had an antitumor effect on the growth of cells by stimulating the activity of tumor suppressor genes, thus turning off specific oncogenes (Diamond). Antineoplastons normally are found in urine and blood but are believed to be lacking in patients with cancer (Willner, 1994). Burzynski determined that antineoplastons stopped the growth of tumor cells, and it has been hypothesized that cancer results from a deficiency of antineoplastons. Much controversy surrounds Burzynski's work and the replication of the findings outside his laboratory. Animal research conducted in Japan demonstrated that low-dose, chemically built antineoplastons could prevent certain forms of cancer (Diamond et al.).

Special Considerations

The National Cancer Institute (NCI), National Institutes of Health, at the time of this printing, is reviewing and exploring the potential role of antineoplastons on cancer.

IP$_6$

Inositol is considered to be one of the B-complex vitamins. It is found in almost every cell of the body, with the highest concentrations in the heart muscle, skeletal muscle, and brain. Chemically, inositol is similar to glucose. The addition of phosphate groups (PO$_4$) produces several inositol phosphates. Each of these has different biochemical effects within the body. The phosphate group may attach at six potential positions on the inositol structure, and this will be described in the name (e.g., inositol monophosphate [IP$_1$], inositol biphosphate [IP$_2$]). When all six positions are filled by a phosphate group, it is named inositol hexaphosphate (IP$_6$ or InsP$_6$). This substance also is known as phytic acid. IP$_6$ and inositol are believed to be synergistic, and the health benefits realized are considered to be better when used in combination than when either one is used alone (Shamsuddin, 1998).

The health benefits of increased fiber in the diet are familiar to all. Cereals, legumes, and nuts contain insoluble fiber in the outer layer. This outer layer also contains IP_6. Graf and Eaton (1985) raised the question as to whether colon cancer prevention benefits are realized from the fiber or the phytate contained in the outer bran layer. This question remains unanswered.

IP_6 is believed to have other anticancer effects, but the exact mechanism remains unknown. We know that natural killer (NK) cells play a pivotal role in defense against disease by identifying abnormal cells and destroying them. One theory is that IP_6 boosts NK cell activity (Shamsuddin, 1998). Shamsuddin also suggested that IP_6 can cause cancer cells to "behave normally" (p. 69). In our culture, we seek to destroy cancer cells, and treatments are associated with toxicities because normal cells also are destroyed. In Shamsuddin's theory, IP_6 is believed to cause cancer cells to behave more like normal cells, which controls the potential for unregulated growth and division. The appeal of this therapy is the opportunity to receive nontoxic therapy.

Additional claims of health benefits in kidney stone disease, heart disease, lipid disorders, and hematology (blood) diseases, such as sickle cell anemia, also have been made. Shamsuddin (1998) suggested that IP_6 offers an opportunity for use as a single therapy or combination with cancer chemotherapy; that is, it provides the opportunity to combine conventional and natural medicine.

Special Considerations

There are no known toxicities associated with IP_6. Individual tolerance may vary. The efficacy of this therapy has not been scientifically proven in this country. However, studies performed outside the United States have provided some scientific evidence of efficacy.

Shark Cartilage

Increased interest in the use of shark cartilage as a cancer treatment is due, in part, to the publication of *Sharks Don't Get Cancer* (Lane & Comac, 1992). Shark cartilage contains a substance that inhibits blood vessel growth; proponents of this therapy postulate that this decreases the tumor's ability to feed itself and believe that this protects sharks against developing cancer (Pelton & Overholser, 1994). However, it has been discovered that sharks *do* get cancer. The antiangiogenetic properties of shark cartilage allow it, given orally or rectally by retention enemas, to diminish blood flow to a tumor, which is thought to decrease the tumor's ability to grow (Quillin & Quillin, 1994) One reason for the interest in shark cartilage is that it does not inhibit normal angiogenesis (Diamond et al., 1997). The usual oral dose is 30–60 g per day; however, doses up to 120 g per day have been reported (Pelton & Overholser). A study by Miller, Anderson, Stark, Granick, and Richardson (1998) did not support the use of shark cartilage as a cancer therapy.

Special Considerations

Any substance to be taken by rectum should be administered only after rectal integrity and blood counts have been evaluated. Shark cartilage is expensive, and many patients find ingesting it in the recommended amount to be difficult. As with many dietary supplements, purity is a major concern.

Bovine Cartilage

Physician John Prudden pioneered the use of bovine cartilage in the early 1970s to improve wound healing (Diamond et al., 1997). Bovine cartilage is believed to stimulate the body's immune system, the macrophages that destroy cancer cells, thereby decreasing the size of a tumor (Diamond et al.). The dose that is used to treat cancer is 9 g daily, and it must be taken for the patient's entire life. Additionally, it may take several months to see any positive effects. It is credited as a palliative therapy, not a cure (Diamond et al.). Bovine cartilage is less expensive than shark cartilage and contains less calcium.

Special Considerations

Purity is a concern, and the cost of bovine cartilage, although less than that of shark cartilage, is nonetheless significant.

714X-Nitramoniocamphor

714X, a chemical solution composed of nitrogen-rich camphor and organic salts, was discovered by French Canadian biologist Gaston Naessens, who considered it to be a promising, nontoxic treatment for cancer, AIDS, and other immune disorders (Pelton & Overholser, 1994). Naessens' research led him to determine that cancer cells require high levels of nitrogen; he described cancer cells as "nitrogen traps." Naessens determined that cells in the body develop abnormalities (which he called "initiation" or "cancerization") every day (Pelton & Overholser). He further theorized that these cancer cells can disable the immune system by releasing a substance he dubbed "cocancerogenic K factor." This factor allows the cells to extract nitrogen from the host cells, which, in turn, allows the cancer cells to grow. 714X is administered intralymphatically. Treatment includes three series of injections of this compound into the lymphatic system, preferably through the right inquinal lymph nodes. A series consists of once-daily injections for 21 consecutive days followed by a rest period of several days.

Special Considerations

Injections of 714X must be administered very slowly. The series of injections may be followed by booster shots. Anecdotal reports of tumors that have shrunk in size exist (Willner, 1994). Weight gain and pain reduction also have been associated with this treatment. Patients who are receiving 714X treatment must refrain from taking vitamin E or vitamin B_{12} during their treatment (Pelton & Overholser, 1994).

The effectiveness of 714X lacks published scientific research, although patients in the United States and throughout the world use it (Pelton & Overholser, 1994). Patients who access this therapy can be taught the injection technique by video instruction. Careful monitoring for signs and symptoms of infection is necessary. According to Naessens, there are no contraindications (Willner, 1994).

Coley's Toxin

Mixed bacterial vaccine, known as Coley's toxin, was developed by William Coley in the 1900s. His hypothesis was that by jump-starting the body's immune system, the body would have the ability to fight cancer. The treatment consists of injections of the mixture. This therapy caused a typical toxic response, including fever and chills, palpitations, and headache. Coley's work was never accepted in mainstream cancer care even though he produced a significant cure rate in soft-tissue sarcoma. The regulatory changes that occurred after this discovery and the advent of chemotherapy regimens obscured this treatment. Patients, however, do continue to seek this and other cancer therapies (Willner, 1994).

Special Considerations

Control of the symptoms—fever, chills, palpitations, and headache—during therapy is important. Monitor for signs and symptoms of infection.

Immuno-Augmentative Therapy (IAT)

This cancer therapy was developed by oncologist Lawrence Burton in the 1960s. He claimed to have discovered a "tumor induction factor" while experimenting with leukemic mice (Willner, 1994). IAT is the administration of antitumor antibodies centrifuged from blood that are thought to restore normal immune functioning so that the patient's immune system can fight the cancer cells. The proteins are given by injection in doses that are individualized to the patient. This therapy has not been confirmed by scientific research and limited information is available. An article published in the American Cancer Society's journal *CA: A Cancer Journal for Clinicians,* however, criticizes IAT ("Questionable Methods," 1991).

Special Considerations

Burton's clinic is located in Freeport in the Bahamas. It has been closed by U.S. authorities on several occasions. In 1986, there was a scare related to alleged HIV contamination at the clinic. The validity of this scare is still controversial (Willner, 1994). As with any "unproven" therapy, care should be taken to gain as much information as possible about the therapy and the practitioner.

Hoxsey Therapy

In 1840, John Hoxsey had a horse with a malignant growth on its leg. Because the veterinarian could not cure the cancer, the horse was allowed to run free and nature allowed to "take its course." To everyone's surprise, the cancer hardened and fell off (Pelton & Overholser, 1994). Hoxsey noticed that the animal grazed in a certain corner of the pasture that was rich in red clover, alfalfa, buckthorn, prickly ash, and other herbal plants. The Hoxsey family, convinced that the plants were responsible for "curing" the horse, developed a therapeutic mixture from these herbs. The formula was passed down from father to son. Figure 4 lists the components of Hoxsey's formula (Pelton & Overholser, 1994; "Questionable Methods," 1993). The only clinical evidence of efficacy comes from John's great-grandson, Harry Hoxsey, himself. He asked the NCI in 1945 and again in 1955 to review his records, but his records were determined to be incomplete and inconclusive; Hoxsey battled with the FDA over his therapy for years (Pelton & Overholser).

Figure 4. Hoxsey's Formula

Tritolium pratense - red clover
Arctium lappa - burdock root
Berberis vulgaris - barberry bark
Glycyrrhiza glabra - licorice root
Rhamnus purshiana - buckthorn
Zanthoxylum americana - prickly ash
Larrea tridentata - chaparral
Stillingia sylvatica - stillingia
Picramnia antidesma - cascara amarga
Potassium iodide

Special Considerations

The dosage of the Hoxsey formula is one to two teaspoons in a glass of water (hot or cold) two or more times daily (Pelton & Overholser, 1994). There are no reported side effects or toxicities; however, licorice root can have adverse effects when taken in large doses, and the original formula contained pokeroot, which can be toxic. (Current formulas omit pokeroot.) Consumption of large amounts of these herbs can be toxic (Pelton & Overholser). According to an article published in *CA: A Cancer Journal for Clinicians,* the American Cancer Society found no evidence of the benefit of Hoxsey treatment in humans and "strongly urges individuals not to seek treatment" with this method ("Hoxsey Method," 1990, p. 51).

Mistletoe (Iscador)

Mistletoe was used as early as 1920 in Germany as a cancer therapy by Rudolf Steiner, the founder of anthroposophic medicine, in which spiritual and scientific principles are combined (see Chapter 3, "Alternative Systems of Medical Practice"). Steiner believed that cancer was caused by a weakness in the "higher organizing forces" that led to excess cell proliferation (Pelton & Overholser, 1994). A commercial preparation of fermented mistletoe, know as Iscador, is marketed in Europe (Willner, 1994). As with other controversial therapies, research is limited.

Special Considerations

Iscador is potentially toxic and can have serious side effects. It should be administered only by a professional experienced in its use. Patients should not attempt to make homemade extracts, as poisoning can occur.

Urea

In 1954, a Greek physician, Eugene D. Danopoulos, reported discovering that urine had anticancer properties. After years of research, he identified urea as the anticancer ingredient (Pelton & Overholser, 1994). Urea is a natural substance found in urine and is the end product of protein metabolism. When crystallized, it is odorless and colorless (Willner, 1994). Older cultures have used urine for healing (Pelton & Overholser). The use of urea as a therapy for certain types of cancer is of interest because it is inexpensive and toxicities are rare.

Cancer cells have a structured water matrix, which produces a loss of cellular contact inhibition (i.e., cancer cells do not mind being crowded). Urea administered under proper conditions and in appropriate concentrations is believed to disrupt the cellular water matrix and interfere with the process necessary for the continued, uncontrolled growth of cancer cells (Pelton & Overholser, 1994).

Special Considerations

The dosage of urea varies according to the route of administration. The oral dose is usually 12–15 g daily in divided doses in capsule form or dissolved in liquid.

Oral urea can cause mild stomach irritation. Urea can be used as a complementary therapy to traditional or alternative therapies. Injectable urea is used in 10% – 50% solution. A burning sensation may develop at the injection site; a local anesthetic may be used.

Laetrile (Amygdalin, Vitamin B₁₇)

Laetrile probably is the best known of all the alternative cancer therapies. Amygdalin is a cyanide-containing substance and a member of a group of substances known as nitrilosides, which occur naturally in plants, and laetrile is a concentrated form of amygdalin. Amygdalin occurs naturally in apricots, peaches, cherries, berries, and alfalfa, among other plants. The Chinese used amygdalin for the treatment of tumors 3,500 years ago (Willner, 1994).

Laetrile has been a source of controversy for many years. Theoretically, laetrile appeared to be a near-perfect anticancer drug. After more than five years of research with laetrile at Memorial Sloan-Kettering Cancer Center, a press conference was called in June 1977. Laetrile was pronounced ineffective in treating cancer (Pelton & Overholser, 1994). Research continued in other countries. In 1978, NCI published the results of a retrospective study of patients treated with laetrile. This study was deemed inconclusive. Laetrile advocates point out that many of the patients had previously received chemotherapy and that the quality of the laetrile used was questionable. Research studies have been a problem. Laetrile was studied as a single-agent chemotherapy, and it was not meant to be a "stand-alone" therapy. Some alternative cancer care clinics use laetrile regularly. However, there do not seem to be large numbers of documented laetrile-cured patients.

One laetrile protocol calls for 3 g of IV laetrile daily, six days per week for two to three weeks. The frequency of the IV administration is decreased and oral administration initiated as the patient shows improvement.

Special Considerations

Laetrile most commonly is administered as an IV. It may be injected into the artery immediately superior to the tumor site, but injections directly into tumors are not recommended. Intra-arterial administration should be done only in a hospital situation by appropriate healthcare professionals. There are no U.S. hospitals offering IV laetrile at this time; it is administered in Tijuana, Mexico. Laetrile solutions have been used in retention enemas and sometimes instilled via a colostomy, while oral tablets are used for maintenance (Pelton & Overholser, 1994; Willner, 1994). There have been reports of accidental poisoning with laetrile tablets. Some patients have reported episodes of weakness, dizziness, nausea, vomiting, diarrhea, and fever after receiving laetrile.

Summary

All of us have heard or read testimonials of miracle cures and spontaneous remissions. Yet, we do not know all that we need to know about many of the therapies described in this chapter.

Pharmacologic and biologic therapies present unique challenges because we know (scientifically) so little about them. They also may represent potential opportunities. In the end, each of us must assume responsibility for our own health, and that may include investigating some of these therapies.

It is important that individuals seek second opinions, validate credentials and training of practitioners, and obtain as much pro and con information as possible before making a decision to participate in any unproven therapy.

References

Altman, N. (1995). *Oxygen healing therapies*. Rochester, VT. Healing Arts Press.

Brecher, H., & Brecher, A. (1997). *Forty something forever: A consumer's guide to chelation therapy and other heart savers*. Herndon, VA: Heartsavers Press.

Bock, K., & Sabin, N. (1997). *The road to immunity: How to survive and thrive in a toxic world*. New York: Simon & Schuster.

Cranton, E. (1997). *Bypassing the bypass: The new technique of chelation therapy*. Trout Dale, VA: Medex Publishers, Inc.

Diamond, W.J., Cowden, W.L., & Goldberg, B. (1997). *Alternative medicine: Definitive guide to cancer*. Tiburon, CA: Future Medicine Publishing.

Douglass, W.C. (1996). *Hydrogen peroxide: Medical miracle*. Atlanta: Second Opinion Publishing.

Graf, E., & Eaton, J.W. (1985). Dietary suppression of colonic cancer: Fiber or phytate? *Cancer, 56*, 717–718.

Heimlich, J. (1990). *What your doctor won't tell you*. New York: Harper Perennial.

Hoxsey method/Bio-Medical Center. (1990). *CA: A Cancer Journal for Clinicians, 40*, 51–55.

Lane, I.W., & Comac, L. (1992). *Sharks don't get cancer*. Garden City Park, NY: Avery.

Miller, D.R., Anderson, G.T., Stark, J.J., Granick, J.L., & Richardson, D. (1998). Phase I/II trial of the safety and efficacy of shark cartilage in the treatment of advanced cancer. *Journal of Clinical Oncology, 16*, 3649–3655.

Questionable methods of cancer management: Immuno-augmentative therapy (IAT). (1991). *CA: A Cancer Journal for Clinicians, 41*, 357–364.

Questionable methods of cancer management: Nutritional therapies. (1993). *CA: A Cancer Journal for Clinicians, 43*, 309–319.

Quillin, P., & Quillin, N. (1994). *Beating cancer with nutrition*. Tulsa: Nutrition Times Press.

Pelton, R., & Overholser, L (1994). *Alternatives in cancer therapy: The complete guide to non-traditional treatments*. New York: Simon & Schuster.

Rosenfeld, I. (1996). *Dr. Rosenfeld's guide to alternative medicine*. New York: Random House.

Shamsuddin, A. (1998). *IP$_6$: Nature's revolutionary cancer fighter*. New York: Kensington Publishing Corp.

Willner, R. (1994). *The cancer solution*. Boca Raton, FL: Peltec Publishing Co., Inc.

Chapter Six

Herbal Medicine

Jamie S. Myers, RN,
MN, AOCN

Introduction

The use of herbs and plants to treat medical conditions dates back thousands of years. More than 120 commonly prescribed drugs are derived from plant sources (Rosenfeld, 1996) (see Table 1), and approximately one-fourth of prescription drugs dispensed in the United States contain at least one active ingredient derived from plant sources (National Center for Complementary and Alternative Medicine, 1997). A resurgence of interest in herbal remedies has been occurring, as demonstrated by the abundance of herbal supplements appearing on health-food and grocery store shelves. Estimates indicate that consumers spend millions of dollars annually on herbal remedies (Marwick, 1995). Bookstores stock numerous texts on herbal therapies, and Web sites that discuss various aspects of herbal therapies abound on the Internet. Many of these resources rely primarily on anecdotal information as opposed to scientific data.

A great deal of the renewed interest in herbal remedies stems from the desire to use "natural" products and to avoid the side effects and toxicities of more conventional medications. However, "natural" does not necessarily mean "safe." Herbs taken in inappropriate dosages or by people with conditions for which their effects are contraindicated can cause serious adverse effects and even death.

The 1938 Federal Food, Drug, and Cosmetic Act required all drugs sold in the United States to be proven safe by being subjected to clinical trials. The 1962

Table 1. Examples of Plant Sources for Conventional Medications			
Plant Name	**Species Name**	**Medication**	**Action**
Autumn crocus	*Colchicum autumnale*	Colchicine	Anti-gout
Belladonna	*Belladonna atropa*	Atropine	Anticholinergic
Camptotheca	*Camptotheca acuminata*	Topotecan	Antineoplastic
		Irinotecan	Antineoplastic
Ephedra	*Ephedra sinica*	Ephedrine	Antiasthmatic
Foxglove	*Digitalis purpurea*	Digoxin	Cardiac
Hemp	*Cannabis sativa*	Dronabinol	Antiemetic
May apple	*Podophyllum peltatum*	Etoposide	Antineoplastic
		Teniposide	Antineoplastic
Periwinkle	*Catharantus roseus*	Vincristine	Antineoplastic
		Vinblastine	Antineoplastic
Poppy	*Papaver sormiferum*	Opium (morphine)	Analgesic
Senna	*Cassia italica*	Senna	Laxative
Willow bark	*Salix alba*	Salicin	Analgesic
Yew, English	*Taxus baccata*	Docetaxel	Antineoplastic
Yew, Pacific	*Taxus brevifolia*	Paclitaxel	Antineoplastic

Note. Based on information from Indiana University BioTech Project, 1997; Rosenfeld, 1996.

amendment required proof of both safety and efficacy. Most herbs have not been "proven" safe or effective via the clinical trial process. The U.S. Food and Drug Administration (FDA) lists approximately 250 herbs as GRAS (generally recognized as safe); however, only six herbs have received FDA approval (see Table 2). Since the passage of the Dietary Supplement Health and Education Act of 1994, herbs in the United States are classified and sold as nutritional supplements (Foster & Brown, 1996; Tyler, 1993). Labeling can only include information about how use of the product affects "structure or function" in the human body; labeling these supplements with information regarding therapeutic use for specific disease entities is illegal. In the United States, there is no sanctioned standardization of purity or concentration. Without the benefit of clinical trials, no data are available to support the most effective

Table 2. U.S. Food and Drug Administration-Approved Herbs	
Herb	Approved Use
Aloe	Laxative
Capsicum	Topical analgesic
Cascara	Laxative
Psyllium	Laxative
Senna	Laxative
Witch hazel	Astringent

Note. Based on information from Youngkin & Israel, 1996.

dosage, preparation, or route of administration of herbal preparations. In 1998, the National Institutes of Health established the National Center for Complementary and Alternative Medicine, which is reviewing the literature on herbal medicines and planning to develop formalized clinical trials to begin to answer the questions of efficacy, dosage, and toxicity for selected herbs.

Herbs are much more commonly prescribed by European, Canadian, and Asian physicians than by those in the United States, and guidelines for herbal use differ from country to country. Germany utilizes a "doctrine of reasonable certainty," whereby reports from general practitioners on efficacy are used (Tyler, 1993). Germany's Federal Department of Health formed the Commission E to review the safety and efficacy of herbs and publish the results. To date, more than 300 monographs have been published (Foster & Brown, 1996; Youngkin & Israel, 1996). The manufacturing processes and potency also are regulated so that standardization exists (Tyler, 1993). Health Canada's Health Protection Branch allows the labeling of "traditional" medicines to inform buyers about medicinal uses and appropriate dosage (Tyler, 1993). England follows the "rule of prior use," whereby years of use with positive effects and no known detrimental effects are accepted in lieu of formal clinical trials (National Center for Complementary and Alternative Medicine, 1997). In France, "traditional" medicines can be labeled and sold after licensing by the French Licensing Committee and approval by the French Pharmacopoeia Committee, and herbal medicines are a staple of medical treatment in Japan, China, and India (National Center for Complementary and Alternative Medicine).

Much has yet to be learned about the use of herbal medicine. Individuals who choose to use herbs for specific ailments are strongly advised to communicate with healthcare professionals in order to evaluate any potential contraindications associated with medications that they may be taking or potential side effects of the herbs.

Healthcare professionals need to be aware of the growing use of herbs by the general public to treat various ailments. While some patients use herbal therapies under the guidance and encouragement of their physicians, many do not feel the need to communicate the use of a "natural product" when asked about current medicines. Others seek information about complementary therapies and their practical use for their individual needs. The purpose of this chapter is to provide an overview of selected herbs, potential uses, and any known toxicities or contraindications to facilitate an open dialogue between clinicians and patients.

Aloe

Common plant name: Aloe; Latin name: *Aloe vera*

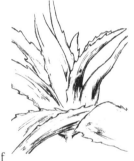

Aloe is a succulent plant that forms a rosette of fleshy basal leaves. It is native to parts of Africa and cultivated in several tropical countries.

Potential Uses

The gel of the plant is obtained from the inner portion of the leaves and is commonly used externally for superficial burns, cuts, and abrasions. In the 1930s, aloe was used to treat x-ray and radium burns (Center for Alternative Medicine Research in Cancer, 1997a). It may inhibit bradykinin and thereby reduce pain (Tyler, 1993). It also may inhibit the formation of thromboxane and, in so doing, enhance wound healing. The gel has been shown to have some antibacterial and antifungal effects and is a key ingredient in many commercial lotions and cosmetic products. The latex or juice of the plant may be used internally as a powerful cathartic laxative; the FDA has granted approval for this use (Tyler, 1993; Youngkin & Israel, 1996). At the time of this writing, phase I trials are being conducted at the Texas Medical Center for the use of injectable aloe to treat malignancies (Center for Alternative Medicine Research in Cancer, 1997a).

Doses/Preparations

Fresh gel from the plant may exert the greatest wound-healing ability. Commercial preparations containing aloe must undergo some form of stabilization in order for the aloe to be effective (Tyler, 1993).

Special Considerations

Side effects and toxicities manifest as diarrhea that may occur from ingesting the latex or juice form of the herb. It may cause miscarriage, premature birth, or loss of electrolytes with chronic use (Youngkin & Israel, 1996). Contraindications include use during pregnancy, lactation, and ileus.

Astragalus

Common plant name: Astragalus; Latin name: *Astragalus membranaceus*

Astragalus grows in northwest China, Manchuria, and Mongolia. It has a spindle-shaped pod with 20–30 seeds and grows in grasses or thickets.

Potential Uses

Chinese herbalists have used astragalus to treat fatigue associated with a variety of conditions and to stimulate the immune system. Some preparations combine it with ginseng. Chinese researchers are studying the potential of astragalus for T cell stimulation and malignant tumor reduction (Heinerman, 1996). It is considered to have immune system-enhancing properties (Heinerman).

Doses/Preparations

Astragalus may be taken as a tea or in capsule form. One recommendation is to drink one to two cups in tea form, twice a day, before meals (Heinerman, 1996). It may be taken daily.

Special Considerations

Side effects, toxicities, and contraindications have not been identified to date.

Bilberry

Common plant name: Bilberry, huckleberry (U.S.), whortleberry (England), blaeberry (Scotland); Latin name: *Vaccinium myrtillus*

A member of the Eriaceae family, bilberry is a shrub-like perennial that grows in woods and meadows of northern and central Europe.

Potential Uses

Bilberry contains a bioflavonoid complex made up of anthocanosides, which have activity in the cardiovascular system and retinas. It has been shown to improve night vision and has been used to treat myopia, diabetic retinopathy, hemorrhagic retinopathy, and macular degeneration (Brown, 1996). Bilberry also has been shown to reduce capillary permeability and edema in peripheral vascular disease (Brown).

Doses/Preparations

According to Brown (1996), one suggested dosage is 480–600 mg in two to three divided doses daily. This may be decreased to 240 mg daily after improvement is noted.

Special Considerations

Side effects, toxicities, and contraindications have not been identified to date.

Burdock

Common plant name: Great burdock, common burdock, cocklebur; Latin name: *Arctium lappa L., Arctium minue*

Burdock is a member of the Asteraceae family. Great burdock root is used in Japan as a food source similar to carrots in the United States. It is a biennial herb with brown, round burrs. It has been easily confused with belladonna root (nightshade, atropine).

Potential Uses

Burdock has been used to treat chronic skin conditions and as a diuretic or diaphoretic (Tyler, 1993). It also has also been used as a remedy for kidney or gallstones (Heinerman, 1996)

Doses/Preparations

No clinical trials have been conducted to date. Care must be taken that purchased preparations are free of contamination with belladonna, which has been reported to have harmful effects (Rosenfeld, 1996; Tyler, 1993). One recommendation is to take as a tea or tincture three times a day (Hoffman, 1996). Another recommendation is to drink two or more cups of the tea per day on an empty stomach or to use as a wash applied directly to the skin (Heinerman, 1996).

Special Considerations

Side effects, toxicities, and contraindications have not been identified to date.

Capsicum

Common plant name: Capsicum, cayenne pepper, chili pepper, red pepper; Latin name: *Capsicum frutescens, Capsicum annuum*

Capsicum is a plant native to the tropics but cultivated in many areas. It has white to yellow flowers that bloom between April and September. The fruit, or pepper, is a seeded pod in shades of red or yellow.

Potential Uses

The active ingredient is capsaicin, which may be used as a counterirritant because of its rubefacient properties. It also may deplete substance P, which transmits painful impulses from the peripheral nerves to the spinal cord, thereby decreasing or eliminating the perception of pain (Tyler, 1993). Capsicum presently is FDA approved as a topical analgesic and may be used to treat chronic pain caused by herpes zoster or trigeminal neuralgia and phantom pain from amputation (Tyler, 1993). It also has been credited with increasing one's tolerance to hot weather, increasing the body's ability to burn off fat, decreasing bleeding time for small cuts, arthritis relief, preventing blood clots, healing ulcers, reducing blood sugar and cholesterol levels, and treating cluster headaches (Heinerman, 1996).

Doses/Preparations

Most applications involve an ointment form of the herb for topical use. Some sources recommend it in the powdered form in one's shoes to treat peripheral neuropathies (Youngkin & Israel, 1996). Internal use is controversial (Tyler, 1996).

Special Considerations

One should take care to avoid transferring traces of the herb from the hands to the eyes or mouth, as severe mucous membrane irritation may result. Capsicum is only slightly soluble in hot water, which makes rinsing it away difficult. For irritation in locations other than the eye, vinegar is an effective remedy (Tyler, 1993). Contraindications include exercising caution in the use of capsicum as a digestive aid as internal use may cause irritation or nausea and vomiting (Tyler, 1993).

Chamomile

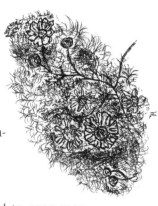

Common plant name: German chamomile, Roman chamomile; Latin name: *Matricaria chamomilla* or *recutita, Anthemis nobilis* or *Chamaemulum nobile*

Chamomile is a member of the Asteraceae (chrysanthemum or daisy) family. It yields a blue-colored volatile oil.

Potential Uses

Chamomile is popular for use as a digestive aid and to ease menstrual cramps. It also is used as an anti-inflammatory for skin and mucous membranes as well as an anti-infective for minor ailments (Tyler, 1993). Chamomile is a popular internal remedy for relief of migraines, hyperactivity, anxiety, insomnia, hay fever, sore throat, gingivitis, and asthma. It also frequently is used externally to improve skin conditions, increase manageability of hair, decrease muscle stiffness and aches, and soothe eye irritation and hemorrhoids (Heinerman, 1996, Hoffman, 1996, Rosenfeld, 1996).

Doses/Preparations

For internal use, chamomile most commonly is consumed as a tea brewed from two teaspoons of dried flowers in one pint of boiling water steeped for 5–10 minutes (three to four times a day). It also may be taken as a dried product (2–3 g) or tincture (one-half to one teaspoon) three times a day (Foster & Brown, 1996).

Special Considerations

Side effects and toxicities manifest as potential hypersensitivity in individuals with known allergies to ragweed, asters, chrysanthemums, or other members of the Asteraceae family.

Comfrey

Common plant name: Comfrey, blackwort, bruisewort, gum plant, slippery root; Latin name: *Symphytum officinale*

Comfrey is a perennial that produces white or pale-purple flowers and favors moist soil. It is a member of the Boraginaceae family.

Potential Uses

Comfrey has been used externally for wound healing and internally for treating stomach ulcers and as a blood purifier. Active properties include allantoin, which promotes cell proliferation, as well as tannin and mucilage. All species contain pyrrolizidine alkaloid, which has the potential to be hepatotoxic (Tyler, 1993). Comfrey-containing products have been banned in Canada and Britain, and in Germany, use is restricted to daily consumption not exceeding 10 mcg of the leaves and 11 mcg of the root for no more than six weeks a year (Tyler, 1993). Like burdock, comfrey products may be contaminated with belladonna (nightshade, atropine) (Tyler, 1993).

Doses/Preparations

One recommendation is to take comfrey as a tea or tincture three times a day (Hoffman, 1996). Others, however, recommend that it should only be applied externally to intact skin over a maximum of four to six weeks (Youngkin & Israel, 1996).

Special Considerations

Side effects and toxicities include veno-occlusive liver disease (Tyler, 1993). Contraindications include use during pregnancy and lactation, as well as in young children (Tyler, 1994).

Cranberry

Common plant name: Cranberry; Latin name: *Vaccinium macrocarpon*

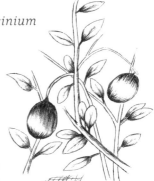

Cranberry is a member of the Ericaceae family.

Potential Uses

Cranberry may be used to prevent and treat urinary tract infections. Historically thought to acidify the urine and, therefore, kill the bacteria, it now has been found to inhibit microorganisms' ability to adhere to epithelial cells lining the urinary tract (Foster & Brown, 1996; Tyler, 1993).

Doses/Preparations

To prevent urinary tract infection, daily consumption of three or more ounces of cranberry juice cocktail is recommended. As a treatment for urinary tract infection, 12–32 fl. oz. are recommended (Tyler, 1993). Cranberry also is available in capsule form; six capsules is equivalent to three fl. oz. of cranberry juice cocktail (Tyler, 1993).

Special Considerations

Side effects and toxicities have not been identified to date. Contraindications include use as a substitute for antibiotic therapy for acute urinary tract infection (Foster & Brown, 1996).

Echinacea

Common plant name: Coneflower, purple coneflower, Sampson root; Latin name: *Echinacea augustifolia*

Echinacea blooms from June to October in the cool regions of southern states and from the prairie states north to Pennsylvania. It is a perennial member of the Asteraceae (chrysanthemum or daisy) family and displays rich purple flowers. Chewing the roots causes a tingly sensation on the tongue.

Potential Uses

Echinacea is said to modulate the immune system by stimulating phagocytosis and increasing leukocyte mobility. It also increases production of T4 helper cells and interferon (Rosenfeld, 1996). It has been studied in Germany, where it is recommended as an adjunct treatment for recurrent respiratory and urinary tract infections. It may be used to prevent or treat the common cold or flu and associated symptoms. It stimulates the production of fibroblasts and inhibits hyaluronidase formation, so it is useful topically for superficial wounds (Rosenfeld, 1996; Tyler, 1993).

Doses/Preparations

Echinacea may be taken orally as a hydroalcoholic extract of the whole plant (Tyler, 1993). It may be consumed as a tea or decoction made from simmering one to two teaspoons of the ground root for 10–15 minutes after coming to a boil (Hoffman, 1996). Some recommend 15–30 drops of a tincture in water taken every four hours for five days, with two days off, for three cycles (Rosenfeld, 1996). Expressed juice or encapsulated dried juice commonly is used in Europe (Brown, 1996). Another recommendation is to treat colds or flu with 40 drops of the expressed juice or one capsule every two hours for 48 hours or until symptoms are relieved (Brown, 1995).

Special Considerations

Side effects and toxicities manifest as allergy. Contraindications include use by individuals with autoimmune diseases and other progressive systemic illnesses, such as tuberculosis, AIDS, collagen diseases, and multiple sclerosis (Foster & Brown, 1996; Youngkin & Israel, 1996). Individuals who are allergic to flowers of the Asteraceae family should not use echinacea.

Ephedra

Common plant name: Ephedra, ma huang; Latin name: *Ephedra sinica Stapf, Ephedra equisetina Bunge, Ephedra gerardiana Wall*

Ephedra is a desert shrub resembling a small, long-needled pine tree. Its needles range in color from gray-blue-green to yellow-green or dark green.

Potential Uses

Ephedra is a Chinese herb that is used for treatment of bronchial asthma. The active ingredient, ephedrine, has been used as a nasal decongestant and a central nervous system stimulant (Tyler, 1993). It also has been used for weight loss as a component of "herbal Phen-Fen" (Heinerman, 1996).

Doses/Preparations

Ephedra may be taken as a tea or tincture three times a day (Hoffman 1996).

Special Considerations

Side effects and toxicities manifest as hypertension, tachycardia, palpitations, nervousness, headaches, insomnia, and dizziness (Tyler, 1993). Contraindications include use by patients with cardiac disease, hypertension, diabetes, or thyroid disease. It should not be used in conjunction with coffee, black or green teas, or the herbs guarana or kola nut (Heinerman, 1996). The FDA issued a warning for use of this drug in 1995 because it can have potentially dangerous effects on the nervous system and heart (Youngkin & Israel, 1996).

Evening Primrose

Common plant name: Evening primrose, fever plant, field primrose, night willow herb, "king's cure-all"; Latin name: *Oenothera biennis*

Evening primrose is a biennial North American native with lemon-scented leaves and an oblong, hairy fruit with reddish-brown seeds. It is a member of the Onagraceae family.

Potential Uses

The seeds produce an oil that contains gamma-linolenic acid (GLA), a precursor to prostaglandin. Its effects may include weight loss, lowered cholesterol, decreased blood pressure, slowed progression of multiple sclerosis, and alleviation of pain from rheumatoid arthritis, menses, and hangovers (Tyler, 1993). GLA also has been found in the European black currant seed and the borage seed (however, borage may contain toxic pyrrolizidine alkaloids) (Tyler, 1993). Studies of a Canadian product, Efamol® Pure Evening Primrose Oil, have shown some efficacy in lowering cholesterol, anticoagulation, reduction of symptoms of PMS, and analgesia for rheumatoid arthritis (Rosenfeld, 1996).

Doses/Preparations

Up to 12 capsules a day containing 500 mg each has been suggested (Tyler, 1993).

Special Considerations

Side effects, toxicities, and contraindications have not been identified to date.

Feverfew

Common plant name: Feverfew; Latin name: *Tanacetum parthenium*

Feverfew has small blossoms with yellow centers and white leaves. It is a member of the Asteraceae (chrysanthemum or daisy) family.

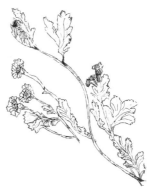

Potential Uses

Feverfew has been used since 78 A.D. to treat fevers, headaches, menstrual irregularities, and stomachaches. Feverfew has been approved as an over-the-counter medication for migraine prophylaxis in Great Britain and Canada (Foster & Brown,1996). The active ingredient, parthenolide, is contained in the leaves and acts as a spasmolytic for smooth muscles in the cerebral blood vessels similar to serotonin antagonists used to treat migraines. It also reduces release of prostaglandins and histamine and may be useful for treating arthritis (Johnson, Kadam, Hylands, & Hylands, 1985; Rosenfeld, 1996; Tyler, 1993). Complete effect against migraines may take four to five months of regular use, and it should be continued for two to three years after achieving the desired effect (Heinerman, 1996; Rosenfeld).

Doses/Preparations

Tyler (1993) recommended the equivalent of one fresh or frozen leaf one to three times a day. Oral preparations should contain at least 0.2% parthenolide. Products in Great Britain and Canada must supply standardized content of 250 mcg per dose (Foster & Brown, 1996).

Special Considerations

Side effects and toxicities include mouth ulcers and uterine stimulation. A "post-feverfew syndrome," consisting of headaches, joint and muscle pain, anxiety, and insomnia, has been reported (Diamond, 1987). Contraindications include use during pregnancy and lactation, in children under age two, and in individuals allergic to plants of the Asteraceae family (Foster & Brown, 1996).

Flaxseed

Common plant name: Flaxseed; Latin name: *Lini semen, Leimsamen*

Flaxseed consists of the dried, ripe seed of the collective variations of *Linum usitatissimum.*

Potential Uses

Internally, flaxseed can be used for treatment of chronic constipation, laxative abuse, irritable bowel, and diverticulitis and as mucilage for gastritis and enteritis. It also can be used externally for local inflammation.

Doses/Preparations

When taken internally, the usual dosage is one tablespoon of whole or "bruised" (not ground) seed with 150 ml of liquid two to three times per day. Externally, 30–50 g of flaxseed flour are used as a moist heat compress.

Special Considerations

The use of flaxseed is contraindicated in ileus of any origin. There are no known side effects if sufficient amounts of fluid are consumed (1:10) (Blumenthal, 1998).

Foxglove

Common plant name: Foxglove; Latin name: *Digitalis purpurea*. Other names include digitalis, dog's finger, fairy fingers, witch's gloves, gloves of our lady, and virgin glove.

The foxglove plant is a biennial. The flowers are red with white-edged spots on the inside. Historically, the drug *Digitalis purpurea* was the raw material used in isolating cardiac glycosides. Now, *Digitalis lanata* is used. The plant is poisonous, tastes hot/bitter, and has an unpleasant odor.

Potential Uses

Foxglove stimulates contraction of the heart muscles and decreases heart rate and oxygen requirements. Historically, it has been used to treat lower abdominal ulcers, boils, headaches, and abscesses. It has been used externally to improve granulation of nonhealing wounds. Additionally, it has been used for cardiac insufficiency. None of these has been proven scientifically.

Doses/Preparations

As a tincture, foxglove should be *shaken* for one day in 25% ethanol at a ratio of 1:10. As a drug, the manufacture of the digoxin and digitoxin is complicated and involves fermentation, extraction, and evaporation.

Special Considerations

Because of a narrow therapeutic range, some patients may experience side effects with a therapeutic dosage, including gastrointestinal hypotonia, anorexia, vomiting, diarrhea, or headache. None of the indications has been proven scientifically.

Drug interactions may occur with simultaneous administration of arrhythmogenic substances. With overdose, an individual may experience cardiac rhythm disorders, stupor, visual disturbances, confusion, depression, hallucinations, or psychoses. In case of poisoning with foxglove, gastric lavage and instillation of activated charcoal are the first steps to be taken (*PDR*, 1998).

Because it is difficult to standardize this herb, the administration of pure glycosides (digitoxin) is preferred.

Garlic

Common plant name: Garlic; Latin name: *Allium sativum*

Garlic is a perennial herb with a bulb made up of small cloves that emit a very characteristic aroma. It is a member of the Liliaceae (lily) family, which also includes onions, leeks, and shallots.

Potential Uses

The active compound of garlic, allicin, has shown antibacterial activity against both gram-positive and gram-negative bacteria. It also has been shown to reduce cholesterol levels and blood pressure and regulate blood sugar (Center for Alternative Medicine Research in Cancer, 1997b). Another component, ajoene, has been shown to have an anticoagulant effect. Preliminary indications show that garlic may enhance the immune system and slow the growth of malignant cells (Center for Alternative Medicine Research in Cancer, 1997b; Tyler, 1993). Initial studies with mice suggest that allicin may be useful in the treatment of transitional cell carcinoma of the bladder (Riggs, DeHaven, & Lamm, 1997). Other studies have associated garlic and other allium vegetables with a decreased risk of stomach and thyroid cancers (Dorant, Van Den Brandt, Goldbohm, & Sturmans, 1996; Wang et al., 1990). It has been used to treat colds, flu, and respiratory infections as well as intestinal parasites (Hoffman, 1996).

Doses/Preparations

The most effective preparation, short of eating raw garlic cloves, is to use enteric-coated capsules or tablets of freeze-dried garlic. This allows the active components, allicin and ajoene, to reach the small intestine, where they can be acted upon by the enzyme alliinase (Tyler, 1993). Dose recommendations range from one to three cloves or capsules daily for prevention of infection to three times a day to treat infection (Hoffman 1996). Dosages recommended for lowering cholesterol and reducing platelet aggregation range from 600–900 mg of garlic powder tablets per day (Foster & Brown, 1996).

Special Considerations

Side effects and toxicities manifest as heartburn, flatulence, and gastrointestinal complaints. Contraindications include use with anticoagulants because of the blood-thinning effects of ajoene.

Ginger

Common plant name: Ginger; Latin name: *Zingiber officinale*

Ginger is a rhizome (underground stem) of a perennial grown in the tropics, primarily Jamaica.

Potential Uses

Ginger contains the volatile oils ginerol and shogaol, which have been shown to possess cardiotonic, antipyretic, analgesic, antitussive, and sedative properties (Tyler, 1993). Some research has indicated that ginger is an effective antiemetic for hyperemesis gravidarum or postanesthesia nausea and vomiting (Foster & Brown, 1996). It also may act as an anticoagulant. It has been used externally, as a warm compress, to treat muscle aches, joint stiffness, abdominal cramps, and toothaches (Heinerman, 1996) and also has been credited with treating poor circulation, cough, arthritis, stomachaches, and gallbladder disease (Tyler, 1993).

Doses/Preparations

Ginger is available in capsules of 250 mg and 500 mg. Doses of 2–4 g per day, taken 30 minutes prior to travel, may be effective for prevention of motion sickness (Rosenfeld, 1996). Use during pregnancy should be short-term only and should not exceed 1 g per day. One recommendation is to use 1 g in four divided doses. The use of ginger to prevent postanesthesia nausea and vomiting has been studied at a dose of 1 g prior to the surgical procedure (Foster & Brown, 1996). It also may be prepared as a tea or tincture.

Special Considerations

Side effects and toxicities are associated with large doses and manifest as central nervous system depression and cardiac arrhythmias (Tyler, 1993). Contraindications include use for treatment of morning sickness during pregnancy and hyperemesis gravidarium (Foster & Brown 1996; Youngkin & Israel, 1997).

Ginkgo

Common plant name: Ginkgo, maidenhair tree; Latin name: *Ginkgo biloba*

Ginkgo is an ornamental tree that dates back 200 million years. It can live a millennium and can grow to heights of 122 feet (Heinerman, 1996; Rosenfeld, 1996; Tyler, 1993).

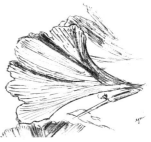

Potential Uses

Ginkgo is used in Germany and Europe to treat conditions of decreased cerebral blood flow, such as short-term memory loss, headache, tinnitus, and depression, and it also has been used to decrease the pain of intermittent claudication (Foster & Brown, 1996). Gingko also has some anticoagulant effects (Tyler, 1993). Other reported uses include as a supportive treatment for asthma, transplant rejection, arrhythmias, myocardial infarction, vertigo, and depression (Heinerman,1996).

Doses/Preparations

In Germany, it is manufactured as ginkgo biloba extract to contain 24% flavonoids and 6% terpenes. Tablets and capsules contain 40 mg of extract (Tyler, 1993). Suggested dosage for use in decreased cerebral blood flow is 160–240 mg daily in two doses. The effects may not be noticed for six or more weeks (Foster & Brown, 1996; Rosenfeld, 1996). Suggested dosage for use in intermittent claudication is 120–160 mg per day for three to six months (Foster & Brown).

Special Considerations

Side effects and toxicities manifest as mild gastrointestinal upset or transient headache (Foster & Brown, 1996). Large doses may cause restlessness, diarrhea, nausea, vomiting, and anticoagulation (Tyler, 1993). Contraindications include use with other anticoagulant medications or when any form of platelet dysfunction exists.

Ginseng

Common plant name: Chinese or Korean ginseng, Wild American ginseng; Latin name: *Panax ginseng, Panax quinquifolius*

As a low-growing, shade-loving perennial of the Araliaceae family, ginseng may be confused with other plants also referred to as ginseng, such as tienchi (*Panax notoginseng*) or eleuthero (*Eleutherococcus senticosus,* known as Siberian ginseng).

Potential Uses

Ginseng is believed to improve sexual performance and act as an aphrodisiac as well as to increase resistance to stress and disease. Ginseng may have useful pharmacologic effects for anemia, atherosclerosis, depression, diabetes, edema, hypertension, and ulcers (Tyler, 1993). Some feel that it increases energy and decreases fatigue. The active chemical compounds in the root are listed as triterpernoid saponins and steroid-like substances called ginsenosides and panaxosides (Heinerman, 1996; Rosenfeld, 1996; Tyler, 1993).

Doses/Preparations

Obtaining consistent products is very difficult because of lack of standardization and some mislabeling of products. Ginseng is available as capsules, tablets, teas, tinctures, powders, and extracts. Because of unpredictable concentrations, most sources do not recommend a specific dose.

Special Considerations

Side effects and toxicities include insomnia, diarrhea, skin eruptions, and hypertension (Rosenfeld, 1996). Ginseng may have estrogenic effects, which can induce vaginal bleeding and painful breasts. Contraindications remain unclear regarding use by women for whom estrogens are not recommended (e.g., breast or endometrial cancer survivors, women with a history of acute vascular thrombosis) (Lucero & McCloskey, 1997).

Goldenseal

Common plant name: Goldenseal, eye balm, eye root, ground raspberry, Indian plant, yellowroot, jaundice root, yellow puccoon; Latin name: *Hydrastis canadensis*

Goldenseal is a small forest perennial with a single greenish-white flower. It is a member of the Ranunculaceae family.

Potential Uses

The Cherokee Indians used the rhizome and roots for treatment of skin diseases and as a wash for sore eyes. Goldenseal contains alkaloids that have minor action on circulation, uterine tone, contractility, and the central nervous system; it may have anticoagulant effects (Tyler, 1993). Goldenseal has been used for oral sores and has been used topically to relieve symptoms of poison ivy (Heinerman, 1996), eczema, ringworm, pruritus, earache, and conjunctivitis (Hoffman, 1996). Previously, it was believed to prevent detection of narcotic compounds in the urine.

Doses/Preparations

Goldenseal can be taken as a tea or tincture (Hoffman, 1996). It sometimes is a component of an "immune booster" herb combination.

Special Considerations

Side effects and toxicities manifest as inhibition of the colon's ability to manufacture B vitamins (Heinerman, 1996). Toxic doses (which vary from person to person) taken by children can cause respiratory failure and death (Rosenfeld,

1996). Contraindications include use by individuals with hypoglycemia, during pregnancy, in children, and concomitantly with anticoagulants.

Hawthorn

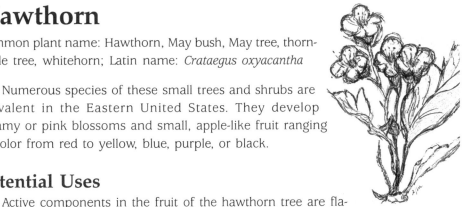

Common plant name: Hawthorn, May bush, May tree, thornapple tree, whitehorn; Latin name: *Crataegus oxyacantha*

Numerous species of these small trees and shrubs are prevalent in the Eastern United States. They develop creamy or pink blossoms and small, apple-like fruit ranging in color from red to yellow, blue, purple, or black.

Potential Uses

Active components in the fruit of the hawthorn tree are flavonoids that have a known action of blood vessel dilation and sedation (Tyler, 1993). Hawthorn has been used to treat hypertension and to reduce incidence of angina attacks; however, no clinical trials have been conducted to date to provide guidance on dosage and toxicity (Tyler, 1993). Hawthorn may inhibit production of a cardiac enzyme, which would explain some of its cardiac effects (Rosenfeld, 1996).

Doses/Preparations

Hawthorn may be taken as a tea or tincture three times a day (Hoffman, 1996). Some sources recommend doses ranging from 160 mg daily in two divided doses to 160 mg three times a day (Foster & Brown, 1996).

Special Considerations

Side effects and toxicities have not been identified to date. Contraindications include self-medication because of potential cardiac effects (Youngkin & Israel, 1996).

Kava Kava

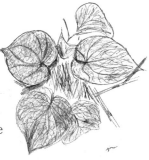

Common plant name: Kava kava; Latin name: *Piperis methystici rhizoma, kava kava rhizome*. Other names include ava, ava pepper, and kawa.

Kava kava has numerous small flowers. Only the inflorescences of the male plants flower. The taste of the herb is pungent, and the scent is similar to lilac.

Potential Uses

Kava kava is indicated in the treatment of nervousness, anxiety, stress, and insomnia.

Doses/Preparations

The usual daily dosage is 60–120 mg kava pyrones. Duration of administration should not exceed three months.

Special Considerations

Even when administered within recommended dosages, this herb may have adverse effects on motor reflexes and the judgment required to drive a car or operate heavy machinery. This herb is contraindicated in patients with endogenous depression because it may increase the risk of suicide. It also is contraindicated in pregnancy and during lactation. Side effects include allergic reactions; yellowing of the skin, hair, and nails; gastrointestinal upset; accommodation disorders; and disorders of oculomotor equilibrium.

Kava kava may potentiate the effectiveness of drugs that act on the central nervous system, including barbiturates, alcohol, and psychopharmacologic substances (Blumenthal, 1998; *PDR,* 1998).

Licorice

Common plant name: Licorice root, sweet wood; Latin name: *Glycyrrhiza glabra*

Licorice is a perennial common in southern and central Europe and parts of Asia, the United States, and Canada. The root of the plant is used.

Potential Uses

Glycyrrhizin provides the sweet taste associated with licorice and is the active compound used to treat peptic ulcer and cough. Some speculate that the steroid-like properties of licorice may be beneficial for the treatment of malignancies, HIV, chronic fatigue syndrome, and pain and to stimulate the immune system and prevent cavities and dental plaque (Rosenfeld, 1996).

Doses/Preparations

One cough remedy uses one ounce of licorice root in one quart of water. One-half pint is to be taken at bedtime. If used more frequently, doses can become toxic after one week (Tyler, 1993). Another recommendation is one capsule with each meal or one cup of tea daily (Heinerman, 1996).

Special Considerations

Side effects and toxicities include the potential for pseudoaldosteronism. Symptoms can include headache, lethargy, fluid retention, hypokalemia, hypertension, heart failure, and cardiac arrest (Tyler, 1993; Youngkin & Israel, 1996). Contraindications include hypertension, cardiac disease, renal or hepatic disorders, and use with steroids or diuretics.

Myrtle

Common plant name: Myrtle; Latin name: *Myrtus comminus*

Myrtle is an evergreen, bushy shrub or small tree. The flowers are medium-sized and have a sweet-spicy taste. The plant boasts pea-sized, blue-black or white berries.

Potential Uses

Myrtol (the active ingredient) is absorbed in the intestine. It can be used in acute and chronic respiratory infections and pulmonary tuberculosis, bladder conditions, diarrhea, and worm infestations.

Doses/Preparations

Myrtle is available in various preparations for internal use. The usual dose is a single dose of 0.2 g, taken internally.

Special Considerations

Overdose of myrtle (more than 10 g) can lead to life-threatening poisoning. Symptoms of overdose include decrease in blood pressure, circulatory disorders, and respiratory failure. Vomiting should *not* be induced should poisoning occur. The therapeutic dose rarely causes nausea, vomiting, and diarrhea. It is contraindicated in individuals with gastrointestinal or biliary inflammatory conditions and in the presence of liver disease (*PDR*, 1998).

Psyllium

Common name: Psyllium seed; Latin name: *Plantago ispaghula*

This plant is almost stemless with one or more rosettes. It grows in India, Afghanistan, Iran, Israel, northern Africa, Spain, and the Canary Islands. It also is cultivated in Arizona and southern Brazil.

Potential Uses

Psyllium can be used for the relief of constipation or diarrhea. When used for constipation, it decreases the time needed for passage of bowel content by increasing the volume. When used for diarrhea, it increases passage time by bonding of water. It also lowers serum cholesterol levels. Psyllium has been shown to reduce elevated postprandial blood sugar levels. It also is indicated in any condition requiring easy, loose stools (e.g., hemorrhoids).

Dose/Preparations

The daily dosage ranges from 12–40 g. Unless contraindicated, one to three teaspoons (5–15 g) should be soaked in a small amount of water and consumed in the morning and evening with at least one or two glasses of water (150 ml of water per 5 g of psyllium).

Special Considerations

Psyllium is contraindicated in individuals with narrowing in the gastrointestinal tract, obstruction or potential obstruction, or unregulated diabetes mellitus (*PDR,* 1998)

Saw Palmetto

Common plant name: Saw palmetto, sabal, fan palm, dwarf plant; Latin name: *Serenoa repens*

Saw palmetto grows in sandy soil in the southwestern United States and produces olive-size red to brown-black berries. It is a member of the Arecaceae family. The plant can grow to 10 feet tall.

Potential Uses

Saw palmetto contains sitosterols, which exhibit a very minor estrogenic effect as well as an antiandrogenic effect. Traditionally, it has been used for mild diuresis and chronic cystitis. Saw palmetto currently is used in Europe for treatment of benign prostatic hypertrophy (Lowe & Ku, 1996; Tyler, 1993).

Doses/Preparations

One recommendation is to take 320 mg per day in two doses (Center for Alternative Medicine Research in Cancer, 1997c; Tyler, 1993). The effects may be seen in two to three months. The tea form is not effective for benign prostatic hypertrophy.

Special Considerations

Some reports of headache, nausea, vomiting, and dizziness have been made (Center for Alternative Medicine Research in Cancer, 1997c; Foster & Brown, 1996). Contraindications have not been identified to date.

St. John's Wort

Common plant name: St. John's wort, amber, goatweed, Johnswort, Klamath weed; Latin name: *Hypericum perforatum*

Native to Europe but common to the United States, St. John's wort has golden yellow flowers and blooms around June 25, the day celebrated as the birthday of John the Baptist.

Potential Uses

St. John's wort is used in Europe to treat anxiety and depression. It also has been used as a diuretic and to treat insomnia and gastritis. An oil preparation has been used to soothe pain from hemorrhoids. Other external uses include contusions, myalgias, and first-degree burns (Youngkin & Israel, 1996). The active compound may be hypericin or xanthones and flavonoids that act as monoamine oxidase inhibitors (Tyler, 1993).

Doses/Preparations

One recommendation is to take as a tea (one to two teaspons in one cup boiling water) or tincture (1–4 ml) three times a day (Hoffman, 1996). Dosage usually is based on the concentration of hypericin in the extract. One daily recommendation for hypericin is 1 mg. An extract with 0.2% hypericin would require 500 mg per day (250 mg bid). An extract with 0.3% hypericin would require 900 mg per day (300 mg tid) (Brown, 1996; Foster & Brown, 1996). Caution must be taken with simultaneous administration of St. John's wort and the antineoplastic agent etoposide. Because of this recent finding, caution should be used with other antineoplastic agents, as well.

Special Considerations

Side effects and toxicities manifest as photosensitivity characterized by dermatitis of skin and mucous membrane inflammation (Tyler, 1993). Side effects with internal use have included emotional vulnerability, fatigue, pruritus, and weight gain (Foster & Brown, 1996). Contraindications include diets containing tyramine, sun exposure in individuals with fair complexions, and use during pregnancy or lactation. Concomitant use of tyrosine, narcotics, amphetamines, antidepressants, and cold and flu medications is contraindicated (Foster & Brown, 1996).

Valerian

Common plant name: Garden heliotrope; Latin name: *Valeriana officinalis*

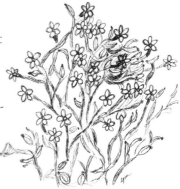

Common to the northeastern United States and all over Europe, valerian has pink and white blossoms on long stocks and a very unpleasant odor to the root. It is a member of the Valerianaceae family.

Potential Uses

Well-known for its sedative properties, the active ingredient has not yet been identified. One of the most widely used sedatives in Europe, it also may be used to treat anxiety, hysteria, menstrual cramps, and migraines (Heinerman, 1993; Hoffman, 1996; Rosenfeld, 1996; Tyler, 1993).

Doses/Preparations

Because the smell of this root is so unpleasant, individuals may have difficulty ingesting tea and tincture formulas. One recommendation is to take 900–1,000 mg in capsule form at bedtime, but up to three times that dose may be necessary before noticing any effects. The effects typically are seen approximately one hour after ingestion (Rosenfeld, 1996). Another recommendation is to take 300–400 mg one hour before bedtime for insomnia and 200–300 mg in the morning in addition to the evening dose for anxiety (Foster & Brown, 1996).

Special Considerations

Side effects and toxicities usually do not occur as long as valerian is not taken for more than two to three weeks without a break. Continual use may lead to headaches and palpitations. As valerian may enhance the action of sedatives, it is recommended that individuals who are taking sedatives avoid using valerian (Heinerman, 1993).

Vitex

Common plant name: Vitex, chaste tree; Latin name: *Vitex agnus castus*

This plant has spear-shaped leaves that grow in clusters of three to four. Its dark berries ripen between mid- and late fall.

Potential Uses

Vitex has demonstrated the activity of increasing the pituitary's production of luteinizing hormone. This increases secretion of progesterone, which is useful in treating the symptoms of premenstrual syndrome (Foster & Brown, 1996). It also has been shown to decrease prolactin levels and enhance fertility and decrease some menstrual irregularities, such as polymenorrhea and amenorrhea (Foster & Brown).

Doses/Preparations

The suggested dose is 40 drops of the liquid extract or a capsule equivalent to 175 mg, taken with liquid in the morning. A recommendation is to take vitex for several months plus an additional four to six weeks after clinical improvement is noted (Foster & Brown, 1996).

Special Considerations

Side effects and toxicities manifest as minor gastrointestinal upset, skin rash, and increased menstrual flow (Foster & Brown, 1996). Contraindications include use during pregnancy and with hormone replacement therapy.

Summary

Nurses play a vital role as patient advocates. As herbal therapy and other alternative or complementary modalities continue to increase in popularity, it is critical to maintain a patient/nurse relationship that is conducive to an ongoing open dialogue. Patients' reluctance to share information about their use of herbal supplements with healthcare professionals may endanger their health. There is still much to be learned about herb-drug interactions. Known interactions may be prevented by taking an accurate patient history. Unknown interactions may be more quickly diagnosed when the healthcare team is fully aware of patients' complementary regimens. Nurses have a responsibility to maintain a current knowledge base about complementary therapy options and to educate patients and families about the importance of open communication.

References

Blumenthal, M. (Ed.). (1998). *The complete German Commission E monographs.* Austin, TX: American Botanical Council.

Brown, D.J. (1995, December). *Phytotherapy: Herbal medicine meets clinical science, Part I.* Paper presented at Bastyr University Continuing Professional Education Program (produced in cooperation with Natural Product Research Consultants), Seattle, WA.

Brown, D.J. (1996, November). *Phytotherapy: Herbal medicine meets clinical science, Part II.* Paper presented at Bastyr University Continuing Professional Education Program (produced in cooperation with Natural Product Research Consultants), Seattle, WA.

Center for Alternative Medicine Research in Cancer. (1997a). *Aloe summary* [Online]. Available: www.sph.uth.tmc.edu:8052/utcam/summary/aloe.htm [1997, October 27].

Center for Alternative Medicine Research in Cancer. (1997b). *Garlic summary* [Online]. Available: www.sph.uth.tmc.edu:8052/utcam/summary/garlic.htm [1997, October 27].

Center for Alternative Medicine Research in Cancer. (1997c). *Saw palmetto summary* [Online]. Available: www.sph.uth.tmc.edu:8052/utcam/summary/sawpalmetto.htm [1997, October 27].

Diamond, S. (1987). Herbal therapy for migraine: An unconventional approach. *Postgraduate Medicine, 82,* 197–198.

Dorant, E., Van Den Brandt, P.A., Goldbohm, R., & Sturmans, F. (1996). Consumption of onions and a reduced risk of stomach carcinoma. *Gastroenterology, 119,* 12–29.

Foster, S., & Brown, D.J. (1996, July). *Herbal medicine: An introduction for pharmacists.* Paper presented at Bastyr University Continuing Professional Education Program (produced in cooperation with Natural Product Research Consultants), Seattle, WA.

Heinerman, J. (1996). *Heinerman's encyclopedia of healing herbs and spices.* Princeton, NJ: Prentice Hall.

Indiana University BioTech Project. (1997). *Cyberbotanica: Plant compounds and chemotherapy* [Online]. Available: http://biotech.chem.indiana.edu/botany/ [1997, May 30].

Hoffman, D. (1996). *The complete illustrated holistic herbal: A safe and practical guide to making and using herbal remedies.* New York: Barnes & Noble.

Johnson, E.S., Kadam, N.P., Hylands, D.M., & Hylands, P.J. (1985). Efficacy of feverfew as prophylactic treatment of migraine. *British Medical Journal, 291,* 569–573.

Lucero, M.A., & McCloskey, W.W. (1997). Alternatives to estrogen for the treatment of hot flashes. *Annals of Pharmacotherapy, 31,* 915–917.

Lowe, F.C., & Ku, J.C. (1996). Phytotherapy in treatment of benign prostatic hyperplasia: A critical review. *Urology, 48,* 12–20.

Marwick, C. (1995). Growing use of medicinal botanicals forces assessment by drug regulators. *JAMA, 273,* 607–609.

National Center for Complementary and Alternative Medicine. (1997). *Herbal medicine: Fields of practice* [Online]. Available: http://altmed.od.nih.gov/oam/what-is-cam/fields/herbal.shtml [1997, September 28].

PDR for herbal medicine (1st ed.). (1998). Montvale, NJ: Medical Economics Co.

Riggs, E.R., DeHaven, J.I., & Lamm, D.L. (1997). Allium sativum (garlic) treatment for murine transitional cell carcinoma. *Cancer, 79,* 1987–1994.

Rosenfeld, I. (1996). *Dr. Rosenfeld's guide to alternative medicine.* New York: Random House.

Tyler, V.E. (1993). *The honest herbal: A sensible guide to the use of herbs and related remedies.* New York: Pharmaceutical Products Press.

Tyler, V.E. (1994). *Herbs of choice: The therapeutic use of phytomedicinals.* NewYork: Pharmaceutical Products Press.

Wang, Z., Boice, J.D., Wei, L., Beebe, G.W., Zha, Y., Kaplan, M.M., Tao, Z., Maxon, H.R., Zhang, S., Schneider, A.B., Tan, B., Wesseler, T.A., Chen, D., Ershow, A.G., Kleinerman, R.A., Littlefield, L.G., & Preston, D. (1990). Thyroid nodularity and chromosome aberrations among women in areas of high background radiation in China. *Journal of the National Cancer Institute, 82,* 478–485.

Youngkin, E.Q., & Israel, D.S. (1996). A review and critique of common herbal alternative therapies. *Nurse Practitioner, 21,* 39–62.

Chapter Seven

Diet, Nutrition, and Lifestyle Changes

Michael Murray, RN, OCN®, and Georgia M. Decker, MS, RN, CS-ANP, AOCN

Introduction

Much has been written about diet and its effect on health and disease. Recently, more Americans are taking nutritional supplements. Many medical experts are reluctant to recommend nutritional supplements, and the recommended dosages will vary from practitioner to practitioner. The Food and Nutrition Board of the National Research Council has been establishing Recommended Dietary Allowances (RDAs) since the 1940s (Murray, 1996). These RDAs were designed to provide a basis for evaluating the diet of groups—not individuals. The optimal level for nutrients is controversial. The RDAs as they stand do not allow for those factors that may alter vitamins and minerals in foods.

Pyramid Concept Diets

Alternative diets have evolved out of concerns about Americans eating nutrient-depleted, saturated-fat-laden foods and a diet high in protein. Jacobs (1996) suggested that, to maintain health and prevent disease, a pyramid diet should be followed (see Figure 1). The pyramid approach categorizes foods and recommends daily dietary intakes based on the importance of the food category to a healthy diet.

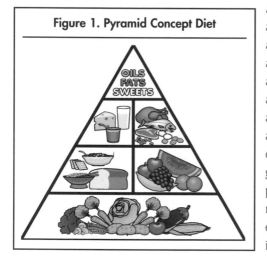

Figure 1. Pyramid Concept Diet

At the top of the pyramid are fats, oils, and sweets (use sparingly). Milk, yogurt, and cheese (two to three servings daily) and meat, poultry, fish, dry beans, eggs, and nuts (two to three servings daily) create the second tier. Bread, cereal, rice, and pasta (three to five servings daily) and the fruit group (two to four servings daily) form the third level. The vegetable group (five servings daily) completes the pyramid at its base. The pyramid diet remains one of the easiest alternative diets to transition to because of its similarity to existing American eating patterns.

Special Considerations

Unlike many alternative diets, this plan includes a relatively high level of protein. It has been theorized that consuming an excess of protein (greater than 8%–9% of total caloric intake) can stress the body's metabolism and that increased fat and cholesterol from high-protein foods may lead to heart disease (Gershoff, 1996).

Exclusion/Elimination Diets

Exclusion/elimination diets involve the elimination of foods suspected of caus-ing illness, gastrointestinal intolerance, or allergy. Suspected foods are removed from the diet for at least two weeks and then reintroduced one at a time. Their effects on the body are monitored and conclusions regarding the tolerance to the foods are determined. Changing one's diet is believed to eliminate or minimize the intolerance or allergy.

Special Considerations

No long-term side effects have been reported with this form of diet therapy. Withdrawal of certain foods may cause short-term side effects, such as headache, dizziness, and diarrhea.

Vegetarian Diets

Vegetarian diets focus on the practice of not consuming meat, fish, or poultry. Some vegetarians eat eggs and dairy products (lacto-ovo-vegetarianism). Research has shown that a properly followed vegetarian diet can reduce the risk of colon, breast, prostate, and other forms of cancer, as well as heart disease and other illnesses (Pelton & Overholser, 1994). A 1989 study published in the *American Journal of Clinical Nutrition* indicated that vegetarians consume more essential nu-trients and absorb them more efficiently than do nonvegetarians (Millet, 1989). Vegan diets eliminate all animal products from their diets. A vegan diet that in-cludes appropriate supplements shares most of the benefits of the other types of vegetarian diets.

Special Considerations

Some vegetarians, because of the difficulty of maintaining a balanced diet, experience deficiencies of specific vitamins and protein. Because animal products are good sources of vitamin B_{12}, vegetarians should incorporate fortified foods or B_{12} supplements to prevent deficiency of this vitamin, which is important in the proper function of the nervous system and in proper carbohydrate, protein, and fat metabolism.

Macrobiotic Diets

The macrobiotic diet has gained in popularity over the past several decades. Macrobiotics by definition means "large life." It is based on the Eastern philosophy of yin and yang, which is incorporated into all aspects of the macrobiotic theory and lifestyle. The basic diet is adjusted for the individual, taking into account the principles of Oriental medicine (see Chapter 3. "Alternative Systems of Medical Practice"), geographic variations, climate, age, sex, activity levels, and personal needs. Christoph W. Hufeland's *Macrobiotics, or the Art of Prolonging Life*, published in 1797, was one of the first books to highlight the relationship between diet and health. Hufeland, a German physician and philosopher, set the tone for the shift in thinking that gained acceptance in the twentieth century. Japanese educator Yukikazu Sakurazawa, writing under the pen name George Ohsawa, developed modern-day macrobiotics. He also reportedly cured himself of serious illness by following a traditional Japanese diet of miso soup, local sea vegetables, and other ancestral foods (Pelton & Overholser, 1994). Ohsawa incorporated elements of Taoism and Zen Buddhist philosophy into the macrobiotic diet. He is responsible for the transition of thought that took macrobiotics from a dietary regimen to a way of life. He saw the existence of cancer as an opportunity to make positive lifestyle changes.

The prevalence of macrobiotics in the United States is due in part to Michio Kushi, who studied with Ohsawa in Japan. He came to the United States in 1949 and became a leader in the macrobiotic movement, founding the Kushi Institute, near Boston, where a variety of programs offer instruction on the macrobiotic way of life (Pelton & Overholser, 1994). Herman Aihara, president of the George Ohsawa Macrobiotic Foundation in California, is another prominent figure in the U.S. macrobiotic circles. Kushi and Aihara both have written books detailing macrobiotic guidelines for patients with cancer (Pelton & Overholser).

The basic macrobiotic diet consists of 50%–60% whole cereal grains, 5% soup, 25%–30% vegetables, 10%–15% beans and sea vegetables, and 5%–10% fish, shellfish, seasonal fruits, and nuts. Methods of food preparation and cooking play a significant role in the diet. The diet can be altered for specific medical conditions, including cancer, and should be adapted to accommodate individual differences, varying climates, and seasons.

Taking responsibility for individual health through a more balanced, natural way of life is the goal of macrobiotics. Advocates believe that a state of wellness is achieved by incorporating the philosophy of the Tao (yin and yang) and following dietary guidelines but also that attitudinal change is necessary for recovery from disease. A major tenet of macrobiotic theory is understanding the relationship between yin and yang and working toward balancing these complementary opposites to create "wholeness." Yin represents functional separation, slower movement, cooler temperature, darkness, and mental work, whereas yang represents functional gathering, faster movement, warmer temperature, brighter light, and physical work (Pelton & Overholser, 1994). Kushi supports conventional therapies in addition to macrobiotics in the treatment of cancer (Pelton & Overholser).

The key to understanding the macrobiotic way of life is to be aware of the continual process of striving to achieve balance between the antagonistic and complementary forces (yin and yang) (see Chapter 3). Followers of macrobiotics believe that illness occurs when the body is out of alignment with these natural forces. The macrobiotic movement encourages analysis and adjustments in the yin and yang to restore balance, thereby correcting for past lifestyles. The intricacies of macrobiotics extend from the multitude of factors involved in determining the relative status of yin and yang. This understanding begins with the individual and extends to the surrounding universe. The diet considers the relationships between acid (yin) and alkaline (yang) and their connections to sodium (yang) and potassium (yin). Quillin and Quillin (1998) identified the optimal ratio of potassium to sodium at four to one. Current review of the American diet reveals a one-to-four ratio. Aihara (1986) attributed the skewed ratios to changes in fertilizers and chemicals used in today's food production.

Food selection also is important. In *A Banquet of Health,* Block (1994) stressed that the selection of basic ingredients should reflect the following guidelines: (a) use whole foods, excluding foods that have been processed; (b) choose locally grown produce, preferably organic; and (c) eat seasonal foods that are appropriate to your climate. Certain foods are avoided, such as potatoes, tomatoes, eggplant, peppers, asparagus, spinach, zucchini, avocado, caffeine, refined sugar and flour, chocolate, and mayonnaise. Beverages are not to be iced. All restrictions are designed to assist the participant in achieving balance.

Few scientific studies exist that conclusively quantify the benefits of macrobiotics. The diet does, however, encourage behaviors that previously have been clinically proven to be beneficial. It is low in fat and discourages the intake of red meat. The use of whole grains greatly increases the intake of dietary fiber, and some believe that this reduces the risk of colon cancer. Macrobiotics incorporates the use of seaweed, which has been shown to contain polysaccharides and anti-cancer substances (Moss, 1992). The program incorporates soy products, which contain phytate and protease inhibitors and are a source of isoflavones, which are antihormones that are thought to inhibit the production of cancer genes. The diet also encourages drinking Bancha, a variety of Japanese green tea containing EGCG, which is believed to protect against various cancers (Moss).

Special Considerations

Special considerations for the macrobiotic diet include concerns about inadequate caloric intake and the capacity for protein deficiencies if the regimen is not properly implemented. The dietary exclusion of meat, dairy, and other foods has the potential to lead to nutritional deficits. Vitamin and mineral supplements are not traditionally recommended on the program. A study by Parsons (1997) showed reduced bone mass in Dutch adolescents who were fed a macrobiotic diet in early life. Dutch researchers also have shown that vitamin D deficiency in children produces rickets (Dagnelie et al., 1990). Another danger of the unsupplemented, mainly vegetarian diet is the potential for vitamin B_{12} deficit. Adherence to macrobiotics can be challenging. Many of the ingredients are ethnic foods that can be difficult to find and time-consuming to prepare. This dietary lifestyle can be exhausting for someone who is ill. Supporters of the macrobiotic way of life suggest attending a week-long residential seminar to assist in making the transitition to the program. It is helpful to have a support person to share the responsibilities of food acquisition and preparation.

Wheatgrass Diet

The wheatgrass diet is one of the oldest therapeutic diets, tracing its roots back to Hippocrates (Rosenfeld, 1996). Modern-day supporters of the diet believe that wheatgrass contains an enzyme that detoxifies the intestines. Ann Wigmore (who died in 1994) was fascinated by watching animals nibble on grass when they are ill and then appear to feel better. She theorized that the chlorophyll in wheatgrass has curative properties and believed that the wheatgrass must be juiced and consumed fresh to obtain its benefits. Wigmore and her followers believed that wheatgrass stimulates the immune system. The diet also includes nuts, seeds, raw vegetables, and sprouts and eliminates all animal products. The regimen incorporates regular use of enemas and high colonics to "detoxify" the body (Rosenfeld).

Special Considerations

Analysis of this dietary program highlights its lack of vitamins and other essential nutrients. It places patients at risk for a vitamin B_{12} deficiency, and the use of enemas may cause infection and perforation of the bowel (Weil, 1997).

Livingstone-Wheeler Treatment

The Livingstone-Wheeler treatment was developed by Virginia Livingstone-Wheeler, a New York University-trained physician who performed cancer research in the 1930s. She believed she had found a cancer-causing bacteria, *P. cryptocides*, and developed a vaccine for it. In addition to the vaccine, her regimen includes a diet of whole grains, fresh fruits and vegetables, and meat. Coffee, alcohol, refined sugars, processed foods, and smoked meats and poultry are prohibited. The use of daily coffee enemas for detoxification supplemented by digestive enzymes and megadoses of vitamins and minerals also are components of the program. The vaccine and diet, however, are only the basic elements of the treatment. The program also includes blood transfusions from family members, interferon, tumor necrosis factor, thymosin, gamma globulin, and other agents that affect the immune system. No difference in survival rates for patients with cancer has been documented (Pelton & Overholser, 1994).

Special Considerations

Past and current scientific communities do not support Livingstone's findings. The use of blood transfusions, the vaccine, and the other therapies listed has shown increased risk for allergic reactions with this regimen (Pelton & Overholser, 1994). The risks associated with enemas are the same as in other programs.

Kelley Program

William Donald Kelley, an orthodontist in West Texas, believed that alterations in the body's proteins could result in the development of a malignancy. He devised a test to measure the body's protein status and believed that the test could detect the potential for a malignancy (Moss, 1992). Nicolas Gonzalez, a New York physician who supports aspects of the Kelley Program, has evaluated Kelley's work. Gonzalez found that by applying Kelley's theory, many of his patients with pancreatic cancer had improved survival rates. The Kelley Program is composed of 10 basic diets, which are chosen depending on the type of cancer.

Special Considerations

The National Cancer Institute currently is investigating Gonzalez's work to determine its scientific value (Quillin & Quillin, 1994).

Ketogenic Diet

The ketogenic diet is designed to reduce the frequency of or eliminate epileptic seizures. The theory behind it is based on the metabolism of fats. When fats are broken down, they produce substances known as ketones. Researchers believe that patients who consume a high-fat diet will have more ketones released into the brain, which will act as sedatives and eventually eliminate seizures. One report indicates that one-third of the patients will be able to discontinue antiseizure medications, the second third will continue to have an occasional breakthrough seizure that requires medication, and the remaining third show no benefits ("A Diet for Epilepsy," 1997). Once on the diet, fluids are restricted and patients are only allowed 70%–80% of normal caloric intake.

Special Considerations

Followers of this diet believe that the diet must be strictly followed or a seizure may occur ("A Diet for Epilepsy," 1997). The potential for poor growth patterns in children is a major concern of critics. Side effects of the diet include drowsiness, vomiting, recurrent infections, and increased serum cholesterol levels.

Hay Diet

The Hay Diet, created by a surgeon named William Hay, focuses on categorizing foods as either acid or alkaline and then combining these foods in an effort to achieve balance, aid in digestion, and promote health. The diet classifies proteins and carbohydrates as acidic and recommends that they not be eaten at the same time. Alkaline-forming foods are to be eaten in a four-to-one ratio with acids. In addition, Hay proposed that protein and starch intake be separated by at least four hours and that all refined and processed foods be prohibited. Scientific evidence has not qualified his theory.

Special Considerations

Side effects resulting from the separation of proteins and carbohydrates may include erratic blood sugars and the signs and symptoms of hyper- or hypoglycemia in some people. Another consideration of the diet is the challenge of maintaining an adequate nutritional intake within the diet's time constraints.

Fasting

Fasting is abstaining from solid foods. It does not, however, mean starving the body or depriving it of fluids. Naturopaths believe that fasts cleanse the system of toxins, improve healing, enhance the immune function, and rest the digestive system. Fasting for brief periods of time (one to two days) may pose no serious health threat to someone who is not ill (Bradford, 1996).

Special Considerations

Prolonged fasts are believed to reduce gastrointestinal motility and lead to nutritional deficits. Fasting, however, is a component of some dietary programs.

Gerson Therapy

German physician Max Gerson developed this therapy in the late 1920s. It is a dietary program consisting of large amounts of fresh, organic fruits and vegetables and emphasizing low salt intake and high amounts of potassium. Thyroid extracts, pancreatic enzymes (digestive aids), minerals and vitamins (especially high doses of vitamin C), and coffee enemas for detoxification supplement the therapy. Initially, the diet included raw liver juice, but that was discontinued in 1989 because of concerns about contamination risks; desiccated liver tablets are now used. Dosing is patient-specific and is evaluated by the physician administering the therapy on an ongoing basis. Variations of this regimen are practiced today.

Gerson had used diet to control the migraine headaches he suffered as a medical student and later incorporated these dietary principles in the treatment of patients suffering from tuberculosis of the skin in the late 1920s, for which he gained scientific acclaim (Pelton & Overholser, 1994). Leaving Germany in the 1930s, he established a medical practice in New York and began to apply his dietary program to the treatment of cancer.

The basic philosophy of the program is based upon the belief that nutritional patterns are derived from humans' evolutionary past. Gerson believed that with the development of civilization, our food supply became less organic and lacked its previous nutritional value. He taught that disease could be overcome by returning to our basic diet. His goal was to produce positive cellular change through diet and methods of detoxification. Participants are expected to follow the regimen for two years. It is theorized that the immune system will rebuild itself and alter the course of disease during this time. Gerson therapy is divided into two chief components, which are summarized in Figure 2 (Moss, 1992).

The specific preparation of food is at the heart of the Gerson diet. Juices are to be prepared fresh hourly using a stainless-steel grinder or press to preserve the food's nutrients. All cooking utensils should be stainless steel, cast iron, glass, porcelain, or tin. Aluminum pots and pans are prohibited, and the use of microwave ovens and pressure cookers is discouraged. Foods are cooked slowly, over low heat, and with very little water. Individuals undertaking the therapy are instructed to enlist a support person to aid in administering the program. With this diet, individuals consume an estimated 150 pounds of fresh, organic produce weekly, at a cost of about $300 a week. The supplements add an estimated $200 per month. Food preparation time is estimated to be 50 hours per week (Rosenfeld, 1996). The additional financial burden represents a limiting factor for many.

Gerson based his theory on several principles that he believed promoted the regression of cancer, the primary principle being the importance of a balance of sodium and potassium on the cellular level. He reported that injured cells initially

---

Figure 2. Gerson Therapy

1.a. The detoxification of the wastes and toxins, which interfere with normal metabolism and healing
1.b. An intensive nutritional program to flood the body with healing nutrients.

The standard daily treatment regimen includes
2.a. 13 glasses of fresh, organic fruit and vegetable juices (high in fiber and carbohydrates and low in fat).
2.b. Organic vegetarian meals, oatmeal, flaxseed oil, and one teaspoon per day of natural, unrefined sweeteners.
2.c. Nutritional supplements including potassium compounds, thyroid hormone, Lugol's solution (potassium iodide), vitamin B_{12}, pancreatic enzymes, and coenzyme Q-10.
2.d. Detoxification by using coffee enemas.
2.e. Additional medications, herbs, homeopathic remedies, or other treatments recommended by a Gerson-trained physician.

Note. From *Cancer Therapy: The Independent Consumer's Guide to Non-Toxic Treatment and Prevention* (p. 189), by R.W. Moss. New York: Equinox Press. Copyright 1992 by Equinox Press. Adapted with permission.

---

respond by losing potassium, which results in increased intracellular sodium and produces cellular edema (Rosenfeld, 1996). The Gerson diet includes potassium supplements in an effort to reduce cellular edema and promote tissue repair. According to Rosenfeld, "a diet rich in potassium and low in sodium increases aldosterone, a steroid hormone that retards the growth of some tumors" (p. 139).

Other elements of the Gerson therapy include the consumption of thyroid extract, Lugol's solution (a strong iodine solution), and the elimination of animal protein. Gerson believed that thyroid extract improved the release of energy from the mitochondria and postulated that the added energy was used to remove wastes and restore cellular function. Rosenfeld (1996) wrote, "Investigators have shown that supplemental thyroid increases resistance to infection, and that added iodine (Lugol's solution) neutralizes the action of hormones that may promote the unbridled growth of cancer cells" (p. 139). Gerson also hypothesized that the restriction of protein would stimulate the production of T-lymphocytes, thereby strengthening the immune system (Gerson Institute, 1996; Rosenfeld).

One of the most controversial components of the regimen is the frequent use of coffee enemas. The rationale for the enemas is rooted in the belief that caffeine, when absorbed through the rectal mucosa, dilates the bile ducts. The increased bile flow is presumed to stimulate liver enzyme production (glutathione-S-transferase), resulting in increased removal of toxins from the liver. Coffee enemas also are thought to increase the absorption of vitamin A, and increased levels of vitamin A may enhance the effectiveness of the immune system in destroying cancer cells (Moss, 1992).

Gerson published several anecdotal reports attempting to support his methods. The National Cancer Institute has reviewed case reports submitted by Gerson, without finding convincing evidence that his treatment methods are effective (National Cancer Institute, 1990; Reed, James, & Sikora, 1990). Scientific data have not been obtained to clearly understand the effects of this therapy. In an evaluation visit to the Gerson clinic in Mexico, it was determined that the control the patients felt they had over their health may have positively influenced their quality of life and reduced their needs for analgesics; benefits of the program were found to be subjective (Reed et al.).

Special Considerations

Astute nutritional assessment and monitoring are extremely important. Critics of the method point out the difficulties that energy-compromised patients with cancer may encounter with the labor-intensive food preparation. Also, identifying a partner to assist with the therapy may prove difficult because of the time commitment involved. The Gerson therapy can cause flulike symptoms in 3–10 days after the method is adopted. These symptoms, which include fever, nausea, vomiting, stomach cramps, weakness, dizziness, cold sores, fever blisters, and headache, recur every two to four weeks for the duration of the therapy. Supporters of the method view these side effects as a sign that the therapy is working. Allopathic physicians view this response as the result of drastic dietary changes combined with the effects of the regimen's supplements (Gerson Institute, 1996). The use of supplemental thyroid hormone can cause tachycardia and other rhythm disturbances. Repeated administration of coffee enemas may result in rectal trauma and cause fluid and electrolyte imbalances. Patients must be closely monitored to avoid complications of therapy.

Nutritional Supplements

Nutritional supplements have been a controversial topic in the 1990s. Theories vary widely, and research continues to explore the potential benefits and risks associated with using supplements. Vitamins are organic compounds made up of carbon, oxygen, and hydrogen. Nine of the known 13 vitamins are water-soluble (B_1, B_2, B_3, B_6, B_9, B_{12}, B_5, H, and C), and 4 are fat-soluble (A, D, E, and K). Recently, a group of supplements known as antioxidants has gained critical attention. Vitamins C, beta-carotene (a precursor to vitamin A or retinol), and E are antioxidants. Antioxidants are a family of nutrients that protect the body by controlling and producing free radicals. The free radicals promote oxidation, which creates energy and kills bacterial invaders. In excess, it is believed, the oxidation produced may damage cell walls and their contents (Weil, 1997). In addition to vitamins, the role of minerals in the diet is being investigated. Minerals are a complex component of the American diet. Calcium, phosphorus, magnesium, chloride, sodium, and potassium are considered macrominerals because of their importance to the diet. Iron, iodine, zinc, selenium, copper, and other minerals needed in small amounts are known as trace elements.

The interaction of vitamins and minerals is not completely understood. Researchers continue to debate the appropriate dosing requirements of these nutritional components. The most widely accepted dietary guidelines among traditional practitioners are the RDAs, which are designed to surpass the nutritional needs of a healthy individual. It is believed that the body's daily vitamin C need ranges from 10–15 mg per day. The RDA limit is set at 60 mg per day, which results in an additional 45–50 mg per day. This surplus of vitamin C allows for dietary fluctuations in intake. The wisdom of this information is challenged by the work of Linus Pauling. Complementary and alternative practitioners vary in their recommendations for daily vitamin and mineral supplements.

Water-Soluble Vitamins

Nine vitamins are water soluble. They are light- and heat-sensitive, and food preparation techniques can diminish vitamin content. These vitamins are not stored well in the body and require frequent replacement. Water-soluble vitamins are usually considered safe because excess amounts are eliminated by the renal system and not stored. However, caution is advised when consuming any vitamin in large doses.

B Vitamins

An article in the *University of California at Berkeley Wellness Letter* ("Preventing Heart Attacks," 1997) suggested that elevated levels of homocysteine, an amino acid, may cause damage to arterial walls, build up cholesterol deposits, and lead to blockage formation. Folic acid, B_6, and B_{12} normally convert homocysteine into nondamaging amino acids, but if this conversion does not take place quickly enough, there is a risk of a heart attack. The article suggests eating a diet high in these B vitamins to reduce the risks identified with elevated homocysteine levels.

Thiamin, Vitamin B_1

This vitamin is necessary to convert carbohydrates into energy. It assists in maintaining the normal function of the nervous system, muscles, and heart and the integrity of mucous membranes. Thiamin is needed for energy production in the brain.

Indications for use include replacement therapy for deficiencies created by alcoholism, cirrhosis, diabetes, Crohn's disease, absorption diseases, and pregnancy (Murray, 1996).

Populations at risk for deficiency states include those who have abused or are abusing alcohol or drugs; anyone with inadequate caloric or nutritional intake for their needs, including chronic wasting syndrome; patients who are recently post-operative; and the elderly. Patients who are taking Dilantin® (Parke-Davis, Morris Plains, NJ) and people with Alzheimer's disease also may exhibit B_1 deficiency (Murray, 1996).

Signs and symptoms of deficiency manifest as fatigue, depression, appetite and weight loss, muscular weakness, and forgetfulness (Murray, 1996). Beriberi is the disease attributed to the lack of thiamin. Rare cases in the United States are associated with chronic alcoholism, pregnancy, lactation, infections, and hypothyroidism.

Food sources of thiamin include soybeans, beans, brown rice, and whole grain products. As a supplement, tablets or capsules should be swallowed whole with a full glass of water; they should not be chewed or crushed. Powder preparations should be diluted in a half-glass of water or liquid to make an oral solution. Thiamin should be taken with food unless one is instructed otherwise. Injectable forms should be administered with caution. No toxicities have been cited. The usual dosage is 50–100 mg daily. For those patients with Alzheimer's disease or age-related mental changes, a daily dose of 3 g (or higher) may be recommended (Murray, 1996).

Special Considerations

Thiamin may produce false-positive urine glucose and elevate urine catecholamines. False elevation of blood glucose, growth hormone levels, and uric acid with large daily doses also may occur. Magnesium is needed for the conversion of thiamin to an active form. Alcohol and Dilantin inhibit thiamin. Thiamin is involved in energy formation.

Riboflavin, Vitamin B_2

This vitamin plays an essential role with enzyme interactions necessary to convert the food we eat into usable energy. Preliminary studies have shown a decreased rate of prostate and esophageal cancers with an increased intake of riboflavin (Guo et al., 1990; Kaul et al., 1987). It assists in maintaining mucous membranes and preserving the integrity of the nervous system, skin, and eyes and promotes normal growth and development. Signs and symptoms of deficiency manifest as dry, scaly skin; cracked, sore mouth and lips; and photosensitivity. Riboflavin deficiency also may cause anemia and seborrheic dermatitis (Murray, 1996).

Populations at risk for deficiency states include those with inadequate caloric intake or nutritional dietary intake insufficient for their needs, such as those with a chronic wasting illness or who recently have undergone surgery. Women who are taking oral contraceptives or estrogen also are at risk.

Food sources of riboflavin include organ meats, whole-grain foods, almonds, legumes, and green, leafy vegetables. When taking riboflavin as a supplement, tablets should be swallowed whole and unaltered with a full glass of water; it should be taken with meals to decrease gastrointestinal effects. The usual dosage is 5–10 mg per day. No toxicities have been demonstrated (Murray, 1996).

Special Considerations

Large doses of vitamin B_2 can cause urine to turn bright yellow. Toxicity is rare and is evidenced by symptoms of dark urine, nausea, and vomiting. Riboflavin should be stored so that it is protected from light and air and should not be frozen. Vitamin B_2 deficiencies usually occur in conjunction with deficits of other B vitamins, and multivitamin therapy frequently is prescribed to correct the deficiencies. Riboflavin interacts with probenecid by reducing urinary excretion of the vitamin. B_2 can decrease the rate and absorption of propantheline and other anticholinergics.

Niacin, Vitamin B_3

Niacin assists cells in creating energy from food. It helps to maintain the normal function of skin and nervous and digestive systems, aids in reducing cholesterol and triglycerides in the blood, dilates blood vessels, and has been used to treat vertigo and tinnitus. It also is involved in the regulation of blood sugar.

Populations at risk for deficiency states include those who have abused or are abusing alcohol or drugs, anyone with inadequate caloric or nutritional intake for their needs, women who are pregnant or breastfeeding, people with a chronic wasting syndrome, individuals with severe burns or injuries, and those who recently have had surgery. Infants born with metabolic abnormalities and individuals with hyperthyroidism and diabetes also are at risk.

Early signs and symptoms of deficiency include muscle weakness, fatigue, headaches, dermatitis, and irritability. Severe deficiency can result in the development of pellagra. Symptoms of pellagra include mental status changes, inflammation of mucous membranes, edema of the oral cavity, and diarrhea. It has been said that pellagra is characterized by the "3 D's": dermatitis, dementia, and diarrhea.

Food sources of niacin include peanuts, eggs, some fish, and liver and other organ meats. It can be formed in the body from the amino acid tryptophan, which is found in protein. Supplements, which are available as tablets, extended-release tablets, or capsules, should be swallowed whole with a full glass of liquid. Oral niacin should be taken with meals to decrease gastrointestinal effects. B_3 is available as niacin (nicotinic acid or nicotinate) or niacinamide (nicotinamide). Nicotinic acid is the preferred form for decreasing blood cholesterol levels. As niacinamide, it is helpful for symptoms of arthritis (Murray, 1996). Adverse reactions usually are dose-dependent.

Inositol hexaniacinate is a special form of niacin. It has the same benefits as niacin without causing flushing and is well-tolerated. It has been used in Europe to lower cholesterol and to improve blood flow in intermittent claudication and Raynaud's phenomenon (Murray, 1996). The usual dosage of niacin is 100 mg three times a day, increasing gradually to the therapeutic dose of 1.5–3 g daily in divided doses. If using inositol hexaniacinate, begin with 500 mg three times daily for two weeks, then increase to a total of 1,000 mg three times per day (Murray, 1996).

Special Considerations

Vitamin B_3 may cause excessive peripheral vasodilation, hypotension, cardiac arrhythmias, nausea, vomiting, diarrhea, and epigastric or substernal pain. Megadosing can result in liver damage, ulcers, increased blood sugars, rashes, and stinging sensations to the skin.

Caution should be taken when administering niacin to patients with gallbladder disease, diabetes mellitus, or a history of liver disease, peptic ulcer, allergy, gout, or coronary artery disease. When not contraindicated, aspirin (325 mg) can be taken 30 minutes prior to the dose to reduce the flushing that can result from niacin. *Timed-released preparations have a greater potential for liver toxicity.* IV vitamin B_3 is to be administered no faster than 2 mg per minute. It must be stored in a cool, dry place away from light and should not be frozen. Baseline serum glucose and liver function studies should be obtained prior to therapy and monitored regularly throughout therapy. Vitamin B_3 can falsely elevate blood sugar, uric acid, and growth hormone levels. Niacin interacts with some antihypertensive drugs and can cause postural hypotension. Lovastatin's concurrent use with niacin may lead to rhabdomyolysis. Vitamin B_3 may reduce the uricosuric effects of sulfinpyrazone.

Pyridoxine, Pyridoxal Phosphate, Vitamin B_6

Pyridoxine plays an important role in protein metabolism. It aids in amino acid synthesis and breakdown, converting them to other compounds or energy. Vitamin B_6 has many diverse functions, including maintaining hormonal balance and proper immune function. It plays an important role in cell multiplication and is pivotal for a healthy pregnancy as well as healthy skin and mucous membranes.

Populations at risk for deficiency states include those who have abused alcohol or drugs, anyone with inadequate caloric or nutritional intake for their needs, including individuals with chronic wasting syndrome, recently postoperative patients, and people with recent severe burns or injury. Diabetics and women who are pregnant or breastfeeding also are considered to be at risk for deficiency. Signs and symptoms of deficiency include electroencephalogram abnormalities, poor coordination, depression, convulsions, glucose intolerance, and anemia. They are rare, however.

Food sources of vitamin B_6 include nuts, beans, whole grains, legumes, bananas, seeds, and Brussels sprouts. Supplements, which are available as tablets, extended-release tablets, or capsules, should be swallowed whole with a full glass of liquid. All forms should taken with food to decrease stomach irritation.

Adverse reactions, including severe nervous dysfunction, have been documented with doses of 2,000–6,000 mg over 2–40 months. In a study that involved administration of vitamin B_6 to combat the effects of premenstrual syndrome, toxicity was documented at levels of 50–200 mg per day (Dalton & Dalton, 1987). Adverse reactions affect the central nervous system and may cause paresthesia, unsteady gait, numbness, and somnolence.

The usual dosage is 50–100 mg daily. This is best taken in divided doses when the total is greater than 50 mg.

Special Considerations

Vitamin B_6 should be protected from light and extreme temperatures. Individuals taking B_6 should be assessed for adverse reactions. Doses of 2–4 g per day may cause difficulty walking because of altered proprioception and sensory function. Protein intake should be monitored because high protein consumption increases pyridoxine needs. Vitamin B_6 lowers the serum levels of phenobarbital and phenytoin. Levodopa's effect also is reduced with B_6. Oral contraceptives, alcohol, and food coloring are B_6 antagonists (Murray, 1996).

Folic acid, Folate, Pteroyglutamic Acid, Folacin, Vitamin B_9

Folate is required for the metabolism of DNA and plays a part in cell division, tissue growth, and the formation of hemoglobin. It helps to maintain the nervous system, intestinal tract, sex organs, and normal patterns of growth. Folic acid aids in regulating embryonic and fetal development of nerve cells. Folic acid deficiency is the most common vitamin deficiency (Murray, 1996).

Populations at risk for deficiency states are those with inadequate caloric or nutritional dietary intake, including people with a chronic wasting illness or who have recently undergone surgery and patients with severe burns or injuries. Women who use oral contraceptives or are pregnant or breastfeeding also are considered to be at risk. Young infants who are not receiving breast milk or fortified formula also may be at risk. Signs and symptoms of deficiency include anemia, miscarriages, and birth defects (e.g., neural tube defects such as spina bifida). A folate deficiency has been associated with cervical dysplasia leading to cervical cancer (Butterworth et al., 1992). Folic acid deficiency has been linked to depression, atherosclerosis, and osteoporosis (Murray, 1996).

Food sources of folic acid include liver, whole grains, dark-green, leafy vegetables, oranges, beans, and peas. Supplements should be swallowed whole with a full glass of liquid and should be taken with food to decrease stomach irritation. Folic acid usually is well-tolerated. Adverse reactions include folacin crystals in the kidneys, which can be associated with prolonged use of high doses. Doses greater than 1,500 mcg/day can lead to loss of appetite, nausea, flatulence, and abdominal distention and may mask signs of pernicious anemia. A potential for bronchospasm, allergic reactions, and general malaise also exists. High doses of folic acid may increase seizure activity in people with epilepsy by decreasing blood levels of anticonvulsants.

Special Considerations

Injectable forms of folic acid should not be mixed with other medications in a syringe because a precipitate may form. All preparations should be protected from light and heat and stored at room temperature. Leucovorin calcium (folinic acid, a reduced form of folic acid) rescue is given *after* high-dose methotrexate, a folic acid antagonist. Patients who are receiving methotrexate should be advised to discontinue any supplements containing folic acid during chemotherapy administration. Folic acid is not recommended in patients with B_{12} deficiencies and undiagnosed anemia because it can mask symptoms of pernicious anemia. If folic acid supplementation is needed, it must be taken with vitamin B_{12}. Pregnant and lactating women require additional folic acid and should consult with their medical practitioners for specific dosing. Aminosalicylic acid, estrogens, alcohol, methotrexate, oral contraceptives, sulfasalazine, and anticonvulsive drugs can decrease folic acid levels (Murray, 1996).

Cyanocobalamin, Hydroxocobalamin, Vitamin B_{12}

Vitamin B_{12}, as a coenzyme, is essential for DNA synthesis, red blood cell formation, and the maintenance of the central nervous system. It is used for the treatment of pernicious anemia and B_{12} deficiencies. In order to absorb B_{12} in food, the stomach secretes intrinsic factor.

Populations at risk for deficiency states include strict vegetarians, anyone with inadequate caloric or nutritional dietary intake, those who have abused alcohol or drugs, and people with a chronic wasting illness or who recently have undergone surgery. The elderly also are considered to be at risk. Signs and symptoms of deficiencies manifest as the symptoms of pernicious anemia, the disease associated with B_{12} deficiency, which include neurologic abnormalities, sore tongue, bleeding gums, pallor, anorexia, nausea, shortness of breath, confusion, headache, and memory loss (Murray, 1996). The elderly and alcoholics may develop deficiencies because of inadequate vitamin absorption. Pernicious anemia is a result of a lack of intrinsic factor in the stomach, which is necessary for the absorption of B_{12}.

Food sources of B_{12} include lean meat, liver, kidneys, milk, saltwater fish, and oysters. Supplements, which are available as tablets, extended-release tablets, or capsules, should be swallowed whole with a full glass of liquid and should be taken with food to decrease stomach irritation. Injectable forms also are available and should be administered as directed by the manufacturer with caution because toxicity may occur. Recommended doses are 1,000 mg intramuscularly weekly for eight weeks, then monthly for life. Oral administration should be 2,000 mg daily for one month, then 1,000 mg daily. These dosage recommendations are not suitable for patients with multiple sclerosis (Murray, 1996).

Toxicity may occur in anemic patients with coexisting cardiac, pulmonary, or hypertensive disease. Vitamin B_{12} must be given cautiously to premature infants. Some preparations of B_{12} contain benzyl alcohol, which may cause a sensitivity reaction.

Adverse reactions include peripheral vascular thrombosis, pulmonary edema, congestive heart failure, transient diarrhea, urticaria, pain and burning at the injection site, and anaphylaxis. The use of tobacco, alcohol, oral neomycin, potassium in extended-release forms, aminosalicylates and cholestyramine can alter absorption of vitamin B_{12}. Antibiotics may cause false-low test results for B_{12} levels in the blood (*Nursing 98,* 1998). Vitamin B_{12} is needed in small doses. The recommended dosage in deficiency states is 2,000 mcg per day for one month, then 1,000 mcg daily. For vegetarians, the recommended dose is 100 mcg per day.

Special Considerations

Reticulocyte count, hematocrit, B_{12}, iron, and folate levels must be determined before initiation of therapy. Potassium levels must be closely monitored for the first 48 hours and supplemented as indicated. Inadequate levels of B_{12} may suppress symptoms of polycythemia vera. Other considerations include awareness that B_{12} is physically incompatible with dextrose solutions, alkaline or strongly acidic solutions, heavy metals, and many drugs. Large doses of vitamin C should be separated from these solutions and medications by at least one hour. B_{12} may cause false-positive results for intrinsic factor antibodies. The vitamin should be stored in a cool, dark, dry environment until use and should be refrigerated, not frozen.

Pantothenic Acid, Vitamin B₅

Vitamin B_5 is necessary for synthesizing and metabolizing fats, for adrenal hormone production, and for normal growth and development. Pantothenic acid deficiency in humans is rare.

Populations at risk for deficiency states include those who have abused or are abusing alcohol or drugs, anyone with inadequate caloric or nutritional intake for their needs, people with chronic wasting syndrome, patients who recently have undergone surgery, and those who have recent severe burns or injuries. Women who are pregnant or breastfeeding and diabetics also are considered to be at risk.

Food sources include most plant and animal foods. Higher concentrations are found in liver and other organ meats. Plant sources include whole grains, legumes, sweet potatoes, and strawberries (Murray, 1996). As a supplement, tablets should be swallowed whole with a full glass of liquid and should be taken with food to decrease stomach irritation. The usual dosage for general adrenal support is 250 mg twice a day. If pantothenic acid supplementation is being used for rheumatoid arthritis, the usual dosage is 2 g per day in divided doses. To decrease cholesterol and triglycerides, 300 mg three times a day is recommended (Murray). Pantothenic acid also is available in a lotion or cream (dexpanthenol/panthoderm) that can be applied to burns, cuts, or abrasions to reduce itching and soothe the wound. No signs or symptoms of deficiency are known.

Adverse reactions of water retention and diarrhea are associated with megadoses of more than 10–20 g per day (Griffith, 1988).

Special Considerations

Assessment of the person taking levodopa is essential because small amounts of pantothenic acid are thought to nullify levodopa's effect. Carbidopa-levodopa in combination is not affected (Griffith, 1988).

Biotin, Vitamin H

Biotin is involved in the formation of fats and facilitates metabolism of amino acids and carbohydrates. Without biotin, metabolism is impaired (Murray, 1996). Populations at risk for deficiency states include anyone with inadequate caloric or nutritional intake for their needs. People who consume large quantities of raw egg whites may be at risk of developing a deficiency. Biotin is thought to bind with a protein in raw egg whites, rendering the vitamin useless (Griffith).

Signs and symptoms of deficiency include fatigue, insomnia, depression, loss of appetite, a smooth, pale tongue, skin disorders, anemia, hair loss, loss of muscular reflexes, anemia, and increased blood cholesterol levels. Babies who are biotin deficient may exhibit a dry, scaling scalp and face. Cradle cap appears to be caused by a biotin deficiency. Deficiencies are uncommon (Murray, 1996).

Food sources include many of the same foods that contain other B vitamins, such as cheese, organ meats, nuts, eggs, and whole wheat. As a supplement, tablets or capsules should be swallowed whole with a full glass of liquid and should be taken with food to reduce the risk of stomach irritation. The estimated safe and adequate daily dose is 30–100 mcg. To promote strong nails and healthy hair, 1,000–3,000 mg per day is recommended. No adverse reactions are known.

Special Considerations

Avoid eating large quantities of raw egg whites because they can decrease vitamin absorption. The use of broad-spectrum antibiotics and sulfonamides reduces biotin production in the intestine. Tobacco use also decreases vitamin absorption. Alcohol inhibits the absorption and utilization of biotin. Biotin should be stored in a cool, dry place out of direct light.

Ascorbic Acid, Vitamin C

Ascorbic acid is an antioxidant, which also are known as free radical scavengers. Vitamin C is believed to be involved in the formation of collagen, a protein-based substance that is essential for healthy bones, teeth, skin, and muscles. Additionally, ascorbic acid is thought to aid in healing wounds, fighting infection, the absorption of iron, and the metabolism of some amino acids and folic acid.

Advocates suggest taking 2,000 mg of vitamin C daily (Weil, 1997) and then increasing the dose when exposed to toxins, infection, or chronic illness. Table 1 lists the RDAs and Simone's (1992) suggested supplementation program. The National Academy of Sciences and Nutrition Board also is developing a list of Dietary Reference Intakes (DRIs), which will incorporate three reference guidelines for each nutrient and food component: the Estimated Average Requirement, the RDA, and a Tolerable Upper Level Intake Level (Blackburn, 1997). Table 1 highlights the diversity that exists in the scientific community regarding nutritional supplementation and is followed by a discussion of specific vitamins and minerals.

The National Cancer Institute acknowledges that while Vitamin C is not a treatment for cancer, studies suggest that foods rich in vitamin C inhibit the initial

Table 1. Nutritional Supplementation

Vitamins	Recommended Daily Allowance	Supplement Amount	NOAEL[a]
Vitamin A (Acetate and beta carotene)	5,000.0 IU	5,000.0 IU (Palmitate)	10,000.0 IU
Vitamin B$_1$ (Thiamin mononitrate)	1.5 mg	10.0 mg	***
Vitamin B$_2$ (Riboflavin)	1.7 mg	10.0 mg	
Vitamin B$_3$ (Niacin)	20.0 mg	40.0 mg	
Vitamin B$_6$ (Pyridoxine HCL)	2.0 mg	10.0 mg	200.0 mg
Vitamin B$_{12}$ (Cyanocobalamin)	6.0 mcg	18.0 mcg	3,000.0 mcg
Folic Acid	400.0 mcg	400.0 mcg	1,000.0 mcg
Vitamin C (Ascorbic acid)	60.0 mg	350.0 mg	1,000.0 mg
Vitamin D (Ergocalciferol)	400.0 IU	400.0 IU	800.0 IU
Vitamin E (di-alpha tocopheryl acetate)	30.0 IU	400.0 IU	800.0 mg

Minerals	Recommended Daily Allowance	Supplement Amount	NOAEL[a]
Iodine	150.0 mcg	150.0 mcg	
Iron	18.0 mg	***	65.0 mg
Magnesium	400.0 mg	***	700.0 mg
Phosphorus	1,010.0 mg	***	
Selenium	70.0 mcg	200.0 mcg	200.0 mcg
Zinc	15.0 mg	15.0 mg	30.0 mg

[a]NOAEL = No Observed Adverse Effect level for selected vitamins and minerals

Source: Council for Responsible Nutrition.

Note. From "Safe Amounts of Vitamins," by G. Blackburn, 1997, *Health News,* 3(11), p. 4. Copyright 1997 by the Massachussets Medical Society. Adapted with permission.

development of some forms of cancer. Block (1991) presented evidence in a study suggesting that vitamin C plays an important role in preventing lung cancer.

Weil (1997) suggested that patients receive 20 g of vitamin C in an IV drip prior to and up to five days after surgery. He believes that elevated doses of the vitamin taken intravenously can improve wound healing and the immune function. Traditional physicians do not support this thinking and believe that vitamin C in large doses (5–10 times greater than the RDA) may be harmful. Continued research is needed to analyze the long-term benefits and potential risks of this treatment.

Drs. Cameron and Pauling are credited with the preliminary research on this therapy. In the late 1960s, Cameron investigated how malignant cells infiltrate healthy cells. He theorized that cancerous cells liberate the enzyme hyaluronidase, which weakens the cell and allows the malignant tumor to invade the healthy tissues. In the 1970s, Pauling discovered that vitamin C was necessary for the synthesis of collagen (fibers that strengthen the cell). They were the first scientists to recommend doses of 10 g of vitamin C per day. Pauling also identified that the production of collagen for tumor encapsulation is dependent on the body's supply of vitamin C. Double-blind studies conducted in the 1980s at the Mayo Clinic found that patients given 10 g of vitamin C did not do better than the placebo group (Hennekens, Buring, & Peto, 1994).

Weil (1997), an advocate of vitamin C megadosing for its antioxidant properties, does not recommend taking antioxidants (vitamins C, A, E, and selenium) during chemotherapy or radiation. The use of antioxidants during chemotherapy or radiation is controversial because of the current understanding of these chemicals. Antioxidants are among the group of chemicals that produce and control free radicals in the body. Free radicals promote oxidation to produce the necessary energy to kill bacterial invaders. Excess production is believed by some experts to cause harmful oxidation resulting in damage to cell walls and their contents. Weil believes that chemotherapy and radiation generate free radicals and that by taking the antioxidants during the treatments, their effectiveness would be reduced.

Vitamin C is being evaluated by the National Cancer Institute for its potential for antitumor activity and its protective abilities against some types of cancer (National Cancer Institute, 1992). Block (1991) presented evidence suggesting that vitamin C has protective/preventative effects on cancers of the lung, larynx, oral cavity, esophagus, stomach, colon, rectum, bladder, pancreas, cervix, endometrium, breast, and brain.

Populations at risk for deficiency states include those who have abused or are abusing alcohol or drugs; anyone with inadequate caloric or nutritional intake for their needs, chronic wasting syndrome, or recent severe burns, injury, or surgery;

patients who are on renal dialysis; people older than age 55; and anyone who experiences prolonged stress. Women who are pregnant or breastfeeding also may be at risk, as are infants who are not consuming a fortified formula.

Signs and symptoms of deficiency include the development of scurvy, shortness of breath, digestive difficulties, bruising, frequent infections, anemia, and slow-healing wounds. Symptoms of scurvy are bleeding gums, loose teeth, anemia, and skin hemorrhages.

Food sources of vitamin C include fruits, vegetables, and vitamin-fortified foods. Extended-release capsules and tablets should be swallowed whole with a full glass of liquid and should be taken with food. As an oral solution, vitamin C should be diluted in at least a half-glass of liquid. Chewable tablets should be chewed well before swallowing. Effervescent tablets should be completely dissolved in liquid before swallowing.

Adverse reactions include gastrointestinal distress that may occur with doses greater than 1,000 mg/day. Many practitioners recognize gastrointestinal intolerance (diarrhea) as the dose-defining variable. They set the daily dose at three-quarters of the total dose of vitamin C being consumed at the time the patient experiences diarrhea. Elevated intake of vitamin C can alter diabetic urine test results, may give false negatives to stool occult blood tests, and can interfere with certain medications, including heparin, warfarin, and anticholinergics. Sulfa drugs, salicylates, tetracyclines, barbiturates, and oral contraceptives can decrease the effectiveness of vitamin C. Large doses of vitamin C promote more rapid breakdown of alcohol. Pregnant women taking doses of 400 mg or more per day of vitamin C may give birth to babies with rebound scurvy. Oral vitamin C may cause diarrhea, acidic urine, oxaluria, and renal calculi. Adverse reactions may result from rapid IV infusion of the vitamin, causing fainting or dizziness.

Special Considerations

Vitamin C should be protected from light and stored in a cool, dry place. Warfarin levels require close monitoring when taken simultaneously with vitamin C because of decreased anticoagulant effects. IV administration of vitamin C is highly debated in the medical community. Megadoses of vitamin C may damage vitamin B_{12} and convert some of the vitamin to anti-B_{12} molecules. Large doses of vitamin C may alter bone growth, cause diarrhea and gastrointestinal upset, or produce rebound scurvy if stopped abruptly. At the time of this printing, the National Cancer Institute does not recommend vitamin C as a cancer therapy or supplement to conventional therapy. Large doses of vitamin C can lead to excess iron stores. Further clinical study is needed to objectively evaluate vitamin C's role in immune augmentation, cancer prevention and treatment, and other diseases. Multiple variables make designing a clinically significant study difficult.

Fat-Soluble Vitamins

The four fat-soluble vitamins are A, D, E, and K. They are not soluble in water and are stored in the body's fat. Transported to cells by the blood and often attached to proteins, they remain in the body until they are broken down. This lack of solubility increases the risk for toxicity because of the potential to store excessive amounts of the vitamin.

Retinol, Beta-Carotene, Vitamin A

Retinol is a coenzyme that stimulates retinal function. It combines with the red pigment of retina (opsin) to form rhodopsin, which is necessary for sight in partial darkness. Vitamin A also plays a role in bone development, reproduction, and maintaining cell membranes and mucosal tissue. Beta-carotene is considered an antioxidant capable of neutralizing "free radical" molecules. Free radicals are thought to cause oxidative damage that leads to cancer (Weil, 1997). Vitamins A, C, and beta-carotene contain compounds called phytochemicals. Plants are made up of hundreds of these chemicals, some of which may protect against some forms of cancer (isothiocyanates) and promote others (Weil). Cyanogenic glycosides such as amygdalin (laetrile) also are phytochemicals. Researchers continue to investigate the complexity of their relationship and applications to treatment. Comstock et al. (1997) suggested that beta-carotene is a marker for protective factor(s) against lung cancer. Vitamin A, in an analog form, and other retinoids have shown promise in the treatment of basal cell and squamous cell skin carcinomas. *Nutrition and Cancer* reported success in the prevention of secondary malignancies in patients with squamous cell carcinoma of the head and neck who were taking these supplements (Guo et al., 1990).

Populations at risk for deficiency states include those who have abused or are abusing alcohol or drugs, anyone with inadequate caloric intake for their needs, and individuals with chronic wasting syndrome. Recent severe burns, injury, or surgery, diabetes, pregnancy, and breastfeeding also are risk factors. Signs and symptoms of deficiency include night blindness, skin changes, weight loss, poor bone growth, weakened tooth enamel, changes in mucous membranes, and an increased susceptibility to respiratory infections. Symptoms do not develop until an individual has had many months of a diet depleted of vitamin A. Well people have vitamin A stores in the liver of up to two years.

Food sources of vitamin A include cheese, eggs, butter, chicken, and liver. Vegetables containing beta-carotene, which is converted into vitamin A in the body, include broccoli, carrots, and spinach. Cantaloupe, mangoes, peaches, and other fruits are rich in beta-carotene, as well. As a supplement, vitamin A tablets or capsules should be swallowed whole with a full glass of liquid and should be taken with food. An oral solution should be diluted with a half-glass of liquid and taken with food unless otherwise directed.

Adverse reactions usually only occur with toxicity. The signs and symptoms include irritability, headache, increased intracranial pressure, fatigue, lethargy, papilledema, exophthalmos, anorexia, epigastric pain, vomiting, polydipsia, hypomenorrhea, polyuria, jaundice, hepatomegaly, cirrhosis, elevated liver enzymes, slow growth, and decalcification. Further adverse reactions include hypercalcemia; premature closure of the epiphyses; joint pain; hair loss; dry, cracked, scaly skin; pruritus; sores in the mouth and oral cavity; desquamation; hyperpigmentation; night sweats; splenomegaly; and anaphylactic shock (Murray, 1996). The usual dosage of 5,000 IU for men and 2,500 IU for women appears to be safe.

Special Considerations

Practitioners should focus on assessing the patients' daily intake of vitamin A and the dietary elements necessary for its absorption, primarily vitamin E and protein. Patients must be monitored for signs and symptoms of toxicity. Vitamin A may increase the risk of bleeding for patients who are taking warfarin. Oral contraceptives may increase plasma levels of vitamin A. Women who are pregnant must avoid vitamin A supplementation because this vitamin has been implicated in birth defects. They can use beta-carotene instead (Murray, 1996).

Vitamin D, Calcitrol, Calcifidiol

Vitamin D plays a critical role in the absorption and utilization of calcium and phosphate, which are essential for the formation of bones and teeth. Research conducted in the last decade indicates that vitamin D may inhibit cancer cell growth and decrease the risk of colon cancer (Garland et al., 1989; Reichel, Koeffler, & Norman, 1989).

Populations at risk for deficiency states include children who live in sunshine-deficient areas (because the body produces vitamin D when exposed to ultraviolet light), anyone who has abused or is abusing alcohol or drugs, those with inadequate caloric intake for their needs, and individuals with a chronic wasting syndrome. Patients who are recently postoperative, as well as those with severe burns, injuries, or diabetes or who are pregnant or breastfeeding also are at risk.

Signs and symptoms of vitamin D deficiency include the development of rickets. Rickets can cause bent, bowed legs, malformed joints or bones, late tooth development, listlessness, and muscle weakness. Symptoms of osteomalacia (adult rickets) include pain in the ribs, lower spine, pelvis, and legs; weak muscles; spasms; and brittle, easily fractured bones.

Fortified milk supplies much of the vitamin D that the body needs to maintain health, and exposure to the sun is another major source. It also can be found in fish oil, salmon, mackerel, herring, and sardines.

Extended-release tablets or capsules should be swallowed whole with a full glass of liquid and should be taken with food. As an oral solution, it should be diluted with a half-glass of liquid and taken with food unless otherwise directed. Supplementation exceeding 400 IU per day is not needed or recommended. Adverse reactions generally occur only with vitamin D toxicity. They include headache, weakness, decreased libido, irritability, overt psychosis, somnolence, hypertension, cardiac arrhythmias, rhinorrhea, conjunctivitis, photophobia, nausea, vomiting, anorexia, constipation, dry mouth, metallic taste, hypercalciuria, impaired renal function, pruritus, bone and muscle pain, demineralization of bone, hypercalcemia, and hyperthermia. A report in *Tufts University Health & Nutrition Letter* ("Vitamin D Toxicity," 1997) indicated that 10% of the people who were evaluated for osteoporosis were taking increased vitamin D (more than 1,000 IU per day).

Special Considerations

Vitamin D interacts with several medications. Corticosteroids have an antagonistic effect on vitamin D, and digitalis glycosides jointly taken with vitamin D may cause arrhythmias. Serum calcium levels should be monitored in these patients. Caution must be used when vitamin D is taken jointly with magnesium-containing antacids (antacids with aluminum decrease the absorption of fat-soluble vitamins), as hypermagnesemia may result. Phenobarbital and phenytoin increase the vitamin's metabolism and can decrease drug effectiveness. Thiazide diuretics and vitamin D may cause hypercalcemia in patients with hypoparathyroidism. Vitamin D taken with verapamil increases calcium and may cause atrial fibrillation. Caution should be used when administering the vitamin to patients with impaired cardiac and renal function. Serum and urine calcium, potassium, and urea levels should be monitored with high therapeutic dosages. 1,000 IU of vitamin D daily may cause hypercalcemia. Patients should be assessed for other underlying conditions that may affect absorption. Vitamin D supplements should be stored in cool, dry place out of direct light, and extreme temperatures should be avoided.

Vitamin E

Vitamin E's mechanism of action is unknown. It is thought to function in several ways: as an antioxidant, as a protectant of red blood cell membranes against hemolysis, and to reduce low-density lipoprotein levels. Diets high in polyunsaturated fats may require increased vitamin E. Research suggests that vitamin E may protect against coronary artery disease and heart attacks by preventing the oxidation of low-density lipoproteins, thereby reducing plaque formation ("Taking Vitamin E," 1997). It also may alter the blood's ability to clot and, thus, lower the potential for atherosclerosis and heart attacks. An article in the *Harvard Health Letter* ("Vitamin E and Immune Function," 1997) reported improved immune response in an elderly population taking vitamin E supplements. Its use in post-menopausal women to aid in symptom management currently is being explored. An article that appeared in the *New England Journal of Medicine* reported that vitamin E reduced cases of prostate cancer but found that it may be harmful in other forms of cancer (Hennekens et al., 1994). The role of excess free radicals in the body is not completely understood and suggests further research.

Populations at risk for deficiency states include those who are abusing or have abused alcohol or drugs, anyone with inadequate caloric or nutritional intake for their needs, individuals with a chronic wasting syndrome, people with recent severe burns or injury, or patients who are recently postoperative. People with hypothyroidism and diabetes are considered to be at risk. Pregnancy and breastfeeding may put a woman at risk.

Food sources of vitamin E include green, leafy vegetables, wheat germ, and nuts. As a supplement, tablets or capsules should be swallowed whole with a full glass of liquid and should be taken with food. As an oral solution, drops of vitamin E liquid should be diluted in a beverage before swallowing or may be squirted into the mouth undiluted. Vitamin E also is available as a topical preparation. Water miscible forms are more completely absorbed in the gastrointestinal tract and may affect dosing.

Signs and symptoms of deficiency in adults may be experienced as fatigue, apathy, inability to concentrate, irritability, decreased sexual performance, and muscle fatigue. Premature infants and children with vitamin E deficiency may be irritable or show signs of edema or hemolytic anemia.

Adverse reactions of hypervitaminosis E may manifest themselves as fatigue, weakness, headache, blurred vision, nausea, flatulence, and diarrhea. Vitamin E and vitamin K should not be taken concurrently because antagonized effects of vitamin K may occur with large doses of vitamin E. As a result, the effect of anticoagulants may be altered and increase the patient's risk of hemorrhaging and thrombus formation.

The usual dosage of vitamin E for general purposes is 400–800 IU per day. If the person is taking a high-potency multiple vitamin and/or extra vitamin C, he or she will not need more than 400 IU because vitamin C regenerates oxidized vitamin E in the body. This results in potentiated antioxidant benefits (Murray, 1996).

Special Considerations

Individuals with liver or gallbladder disease must be monitored for response to vitamin E therapy. These organs affect bile production, which is essential for vitamin E absorption. Medications also can affect vitamin absorption. Excessive doses of vitamin E cause vitamin A depletion. Tobacco decreases absorption, and chronic alcoholism diminishes vitamin E stores in the liver. Supplements should be stored in a cool, dry place, avoiding exposure to light and extreme temperatures. Water-miscible forms of the vitamin are more completely absorbed in the gastrointestinal tract, which may affect dosing.

Menadiol, Phytonadione (Aquamephyton), Vitamin K

Vitamin K's primary role is the manufacture of clotting factors. It promotes normal growth and development, prevents hemorrhagic disease in newborns, is necessary in the formation of proteins vital for blood clotting, and is used in the treatment of bleeding disorders caused by vitamin K deficiencies. Vitamin K is necessary for allowing osteocalcin (a noncollagen protein found in bones) to join with calcium, resulting in calcium retention within bone (Murray, 1996).

Deficiency states are rare, but those populations at risk include people who are abusing or have abused alcohol, anyone with inadequate caloric or nutritional intake for their needs, diabetics, patients who are recently postoperative, and premature infants. People with recent severe burns or injury also are at risk, as are individuals who are taking antibiotics that may destroy normal intestinal flora needed to produce vitamin K and those who do not have adequate bile to absorb fats.

Signs and symptoms of deficiency in adults include abnormal blood clotting (which may exhibit as nosebleeds), blood in the urine, gastric bleeding, or bruising. Hemorrhagic disease in newborns is characterized by intestinal bleeding and vomiting blood. Bleeding can occur from the umbilical cord or circumcision site. Symptoms begin within two to three days after birth.

Food sources of vitamin K include dark-green, leafy vegetables, broccoli, Brussels sprouts, liver, egg yolks, and herbal and green tea. Vitamin K also is produced in the intestines when normal flora are present. As a supplement, tablets should be swallowed whole with a full glass of liquid and should be taken with food. Vitamin K also may be administered intravenously, subcutaneously, or intramuscularly (individuals should consult the package insert for administration route restrictions). Administration routes and dosing vary between adults and pediatric populations. Prudent administration is necessary to avoid side effects and reactions.

Adverse reactions often are associated with sensitivity reactions, rapid infusion, and megadosing. Adverse reactions can present in infants as hemolytic anemia, hyberbilirubinemia, or jaundice and in adults as dizziness, a rapid and weak pulse, transient hypotension, diaphoresis, and flushing; erythema, pain, hematoma, and swelling at injection site; and anaphylaxis (*Nursing 98,* 1998). Vitamin K may counteract anticoagulant drugs such as warfarin.

The best supplementation plan is to increase the intake of green, leafy vegetables and take 150–500 mcg of vitamin K. K_1 is the preferred form for oral supplementation. One of the best sources of K_1 is chlorophyll. The natural chlorophyll that occurs in plants is fat soluble. Most oral chlorophyll supplements are water soluble.

Special Considerations

Individuals who are taking vitamin K and anticoagulants should be monitored for interactions. Recommended guidelines should be followed to ensure safe delivery of therapy. Vitamin K should be protected from exposure to light. Individuals should be monitored for coagulation irregularities and assessed for sensitivity reactions.

Minerals

Minerals are inorganic nutrients that participate in protein synthesis and the balancing of body fluids and act as catalysts for cellular functions. The body requires larger amounts of the major minerals (i.e., calcium, phosphorus, magnesium, sodium, potassium, chloride, and sulfur) than the trace minerals (i.e., chromium, copper, iodine, iron, manganese, molybdenum, selenium, zinc, boron, silicon, and vanadium). RDAs have been established for calcium, magnesium, phosphorus, iron, iodine, selenium, and zinc. All mineral supplements should be stored in a cool, dry location out of direct light and protected from extreme temperatures.

Calcium

Calcium is essential to the development and maintenance of bones and teeth. Muscle contraction, neurotransmitter release, regulation of heartbeat, and blood clotting require calcium. It is the most abundant mineral in the human body, making up 1.5%–2% of total body weight. More than 99% of the body's calcium is contained in the bones.

Populations at risk for deficiency states include those with lactose intolerance, on a high-protein nutritional program (which increases urinary excretion of calcium), or receiving thyroid replacement therapy. Individuals with a small build, prematurely graying hair, family history of calcium deficiency, and poor nutritional history also are at risk. Additional factors for women include being postmenopausal, white or Asian, or prematurely menopausal and having sedentary lifestyle. Long-term use of anticonvulsants, gastric or small bowel resection, long-term steroid use, smoking, and history of alcohol abuse also can contribute to calcium deficiency. The usual dosage of calcium as a supplement is 1,000 mg daily for adults. For pregnant women and during lactation, 1,200 mg per day is recommended. For postmenopausal women, 1,500 mg daily is the optimal dose.

Signs and symptoms of deficiency include osteopenia or bone loss as seen via DEXA scan or the equivalent. Deficiency states in children include rickets. Osteomalacia may result from calcium deficiency. Low blood levels may exhibit as muscle and leg cramps. Inadequate intake can contribute to high blood pressure and colon cancer.

Food sources include primarily dairy products, although spinach, kale, turnips, collard greens, mustard greens, broccoli, and tofu are excellent sources. Carob flour, almonds, sunflower seeds, raisins, brown rice, and dried prunes also are good sources. As a supplement, calcium tablets should be swallowed whole with water. Simultaneous consumption with tea, coffee, dairy products, spinach, rhubarb, bran, whole-grain cereals, fresh fruit, and vegetables should be avoided because these substances can interfere with absorption and utilization of the supplement. Calcium supplements vary in dosage from brand to brand. Some preparations also contain vitamin D, which is needed for absorption.

Adverse reactions, particularly development of kidney stones, may be associated with doses in excess of 2,500 mg per day. Severe nausea, vomiting, low blood sugar, muscle weakness, difficulty breathing, and arrhythmias may signal impending toxicity.

The recommended dose for adults, including premenopausal women, is 1,000 mg of elemental calcium per day and for postmenopausal women is 1,500 mg per day (actual requirements may vary with individual differences). Patients with cancer or hyperparathyroidism should only take calcium supplements under the supervision of a healthcare provider.

Special Considerations

All supplements that an individual is taking should be evaluated. Should other supplements contain vitamin D, the individual may not require additional vitamin D in a calcium preparation. Calcium preparations also may contain magnesium. Patient education must include information regarding foods and beverages that may interfere with calcium absorption and on the signs and symptoms of overdose. Dietary protein and dairy intake should be assessed in all men and women. Patients who are receiving thyroid replacement therapy may require additional calcium and magnesium. Appropriate follow-up with DEXA scan or the equivalent is essential. A few machines that measure bone density by calculating the values at the ankle or wrist are available. These are less expensive and reasonably accurate.

Potassium

Potassium is a mineral salt that has the potential to conduct electricity. It is closely related to sodium and chloride in function. Sodium-to-potassium ratio should be one to five to maintain health. The average American diet usually is much higher in sodium than potassium.

Populations at risk for deficiency states include the elderly, individuals who take diuretics or laxatives, and those with high blood pressure. Because potassium is excreted in sweat, athletes are at risk for deficiency states. Signs and symptoms of deficiency manifest as fatigue, irritability, weakness, heart irregularities, muscle weakness, and an alteration in nerve conduction. A diet high in potassium and low in fruits and vegetables can cause a potassium deficiency.

Food sources of potassium include fresh vegetables, fresh fruit, and unprocessed meats and fish. The FDA controls the amount of potassium available in non-food-based forms. Salt substitutes actually are potassium chloride. Potassium chloride is available by prescription, as well.

Adverse reactions to potassium salts include nausea, vomiting, and diarrhea when consumed in pill form at increased dosages. No adverse reactions are noted from potassium consumed as food or food-based supplements except in those with kidney disease, who usually need to restrict their potassium intake. Potassium supplements are contraindicated in individuals who take certain medications, including digitalis, potassium-sparing diuretics, and angiotensin-converting enzyme (ACE) inhibitors. A safe and adequate intake of potassium is 1.9–5.6 g.

Special Considerations

Deficiency-inducing situations and contraindications should be avoided. People with kidney disease cannot handle a potassium excess; therefore, their potassium usually is restricted.

Magnesium

Magnesium is second to potassium in concentration in the cells of the body. The bones contain more than half of the body's magnesium content. The highest concentrations of this mineral are in the brain, heart, liver, and kidneys.

Magnesium deficiency usually results from inadequate absorption or increased excretion. Populations at risk for deficiency states include primarily the elderly and anyone with a decreased nutritional status or impaired intestinal absorption. It also has been noted in women during the premenstrual period. Other at-risk populations include individuals who have a high calcium intake, those who are abusing or have abused alcohol, patients who are recently postoperative, those who regularly use diuretics, patients with liver or kidney disease, and women who take birth control pills. Conditions associated with a magnesium deficiency include acute pancreatitis, high blood pressure, congestive heart failure, digitalis toxicity, kidney stones, and impaired absorption by the intestines. Magnesium has been referred to as a natural calcium channel blocker. Signs and symptoms of deficiency include fatigue, mental confusion, irritability, weakness and problems in muscle contraction, muscle cramps, anorexia, insomnia, and problems in nerve conduction (Murray, 1996).

Food sources of magnesium include tofu, legumes, seeds, nuts, whole grains, and green, leafy vegetables. Refined foods, meat, and dairy products are low in magnesium. Magnesium supplements are available in several forms, all of which are readily absorbed. Dosage ranges vary from 6 mg/kg of body weight to 12 mg/kg of body weight per day. The higher doses usually are recommended when some of the conditions associated with deficiency exist.

Adverse reactions can occur in individuals with kidney disease or severe heart disease. In these cases, magnesium supplements should not be taken without appropriate supervision. Many drugs adversely affect magnesium status, including diuretics, insulin, and digitalis.

Special Considerations

Patients should be evaluated for factors that interfere with magnesium absorption and assessed for potential benefits of magnesium supplements. Deficiency states can be evaluated by examining magnesium concentrations in red blood cells.

Chromium

Chromium has been touted as a treatment for a number of health conditions. Chromium has been marketed as the supplement that can aid in weight loss, improve sexual function, and boost energy. Its primary effect is on blood sugar control.

Populations at risk for deficiency states include those with impaired glucose tolerance and elevated cholesterol and triglyceride levels. It is being studied as an acne treatment (Murray, 1996). Signs and symptoms of deficiency primarily present as glucose intolerance, as evidenced by elevated blood sugar and insulin levels. The primary use of chromium supplementation is for impaired glucose tolerance (diabetes and hypoglycemia).

Food sources of chromium are meats and whole grains. Fruits, vegetables, and dairy products are low in chromium. It is suggested that at least 200 mcg are needed per day. Some practitioners recommend 400–600 mcg per day during/for weight loss. No adverse reactions have been reported, although an interesting reported side effect is an increase in dream activity when chromium is taken in the evening (Murray, 1996).

Special Considerations

White flour and refined sugar should be avoided, as they may deplete chromium levels in the body. Lack of exercise also depletes chromium levels. Antacids may interfere with chromium absorption. Supplementation can be considered in individuals who have impaired glucose tolerance or elevated cholesterol and triglycerides.

Copper

The third most plentiful essential trace mineral, copper is involved in key chemical reactions in the body. The highest concentrations occur in the brain and liver, while the greatest amount occurs in skeletal muscle, but it also is present in bone, skin, and bone marrow.

Populations at risk for deficiencies include people with inadequate nutritional intake, individuals with impaired absorption, those who are receiving chelation therapy and other loss states, and those with increased requirement secondary to pregnancy and breastfeeding. Individuals who take zinc supplements also are at risk for deficiency states.

Signs and symptoms of deficiency states occur when the system reactions that require copper do not occur or are altered. Copper deficiency manifests as poor collagen integrity including rupture of blood vessels, osteoporosis, bone and joint changes, elevated low-density lipoprotein and decreased high-density lipoprotein, and brain disturbances.

Food sources of copper include oysters, other shellfish, legumes, olive oil, almonds, hazelnuts, walnuts, pecans, barley, whole wheat, and coconut. Many supplement forms are available, but whether one is better than another is unknown. Safe intake is considered to be 1.3–3.0 mg per day. Adverse reactions include nausea and vomiting. Toxicity is rare (Murray, 1996).

Special Considerations

Copper intake can have a negative impact on zinc levels in the body, and vitamin C, iron, and other minerals can inhibit copper absorption. Copper bracelets are popular for pain relief in the treatment of arthritis; some scientific support for this exists (Weil, 1997).

Iodine

Iodine is a trace element that is needed for the creation of thyroid hormone. Populations at risk for deficiency include those who use sea salt as opposed to table salt, which is fortified with iodine. Iodine deficiency can be especially problematic in women who are pregnant and in fetal development. Signs and symptoms of deficiency states include goiter, growth retardation, early- and late-pregnancy miscarriage, and cretinism.

Food sources of iodine include seafood and kelp. In the United States, iodized salt is the most common dietary source. When elemental iodine is complexed to sodium or potassium, it becomes an iodide. The body uses iodine and iodide differently. Iodide has a stronger effect on thyroid function, whereas iodine has a stronger effect on other functions. The RDA of iodine is less than 500 mcg.

Adverse reactions manifest as impaired thyroid hormone when oral administration exceeds 500 mcg/day. Increased dietary intake is associated with acne-like skin reactions. No drug reactions are known.

Special Considerations

Individuals should be monitored for the signs and symptoms of deficiency states.

Iron

Iron is essential for human life. It is necessary for the manufacture of hemoglobin, the key molecule in red blood cells responsible for the transport of oxygen from the lungs to body tissues. Iron deficiency is the most common nutrient deficiency in the United States (Murray, 1996).

Populations at risk for deficiency states include infants, teenage girls, and pregnant women. Anyone in these groups or with decreased absorption or blood loss is at risk. Elderly individuals also are at risk because of insufficient dietary intake and decreased absorption. Signs and symptoms of deficiency manifest as impaired oxygen delivery, anemia, impaired immune function, menstrual abnormalities, and decreased energy.

Food sources of iron include kelp, Brewer's yeast, wheat bran, liver, beef, sunflower seeds, almonds, dried prunes, beans, tofu, broccoli, and millet. As a supplement, 30 mg of iron succinate or furmarate is recommended twice a day between meals to promote absorption. If this causes gastrointestinal discomfort, 30 mg can be taken three times a day with meals.

Adverse reactions may include an increased risk of heart disease with high iron levels. Vitamins C and E are believed to protect against this risk (Murray, 1996). Iron overload has been associated with increased risk of infection. Iron poisoning exhibits as nausea, vomiting, and shock and results in intestinal and liver damage.

Special Considerations

Individuals should be monitored for deficiency states. Iron-deficiency anemia is late-stage iron deficiency. Serum ferritin is the best laboratory assessment of iron stores in the body. Acute iron poisoning can occur in children. Therefore, iron supplements should be stored out of the reach of children.

Manganese

Manganese is essential for growth and reproduction. Populations at risk for deficiency states include babies born to women who are in a deficiency state during pregnancy. The major indications for supplementation include strains, sprains, and inflammation.

Signs and symptoms of deficiency states are not well-defined but include metabolic disturbances, skin rash, and hair and nail changes. Babies born to mothers with a deficiency exhibit ataxia.

Food sources of manganese include pecans, Brazil nuts, almonds, barley, rye, buckwheat, split peas, spinach, oats and oatmeal, peanuts, raisins, Brussels sprouts, cornmeal, brown rice, carrots, and broccoli, as well as meats, dairy products, and poultry. While no official supplement dosage has been recommended, dosages of 2.5–5.0 mg per day for adults are considered to be safe. For the treatment of strains and sprains, 50–200 mg per day should be taken in divided doses, then decreased. Manganese salts are thought to be less well-absorbed than manganese picolinate or gluconate; however, this has not been scientifically substantiated.

Adverse reactions include "manganese madness," which presents as hallucinations, violent behavior, and hyperirritability. This is rare and usually a result of environmental pollution (Murray, 1996).

Special Considerations

Certain supplements interfere in manganese absorption (i.e., magnesium, calcium, iron, copper, and zinc). Antacids also may inhibit absorption. Manganese is a cofactor in glucose metabolism. Low manganese has been associated with epilepsy.

Selenium

Selenium is a trace mineral that functions as an antioxidant. Low selenium levels are associated with an increased risk for some cancers, cardiovascular disease, and inflammatory conditions (Murray, 1996). Low levels of this trace mineral also have been associated with cataract formation. Selenium is an antagonist to heavy metals, such as lead, mercury, aluminum, and cadmium.

Populations at risk for deficiency states include those who are receiving cancer chemotherapy; individuals who are exposed to cadmium, lead, mercury, and other heavy metals; and people who are taking zinc supplements. Signs and symptoms of deficiency are rare but include muscle weakness and heart disturbances. Chronically low selenium intake is associated with an increased risk for cancer, heart disease, and low immune system function (Murray, 1996).

Food sources include wheat germ, Brazil nuts, oats, bran, barley, orange juice, garlic, brown rice, and whole wheat. As a supplement, selenium is available in several forms. Inorganic salts (sodium selenite) are not as effectively absorbed as organic forms (high-selenium-content yeast).

Adverse reactions include hair loss, horizontal streaking of nails, intermittent nausea and vomiting, fatigue, and "sour milk" breath with large doses over time. Toxicity is rare. Sustained elevated selenium levels have been associated with dental caries (Murray, 1996).

Special Considerations

No RDA for selenium has been established. For adults, 50–200 mcg per day is the recommended dosage range. Some research has indicated a dose of 200 mcg per day to reduce the risk of colon cancer.

Zinc

Zinc is the second most abundant trace mineral in the body. Zinc is necessary for the action of thymic hormones, insulin, and growth hormone, which promote normal growth and development

Populations at risk for deficiency states include pregnant and breastfeeding women, vegetarians, athletes, those who are or have been abusing alcohol, elderly individuals, those with a history of "crash" dieting or starvation, patients who have sustained trauma, patients who are receiving dialysis, and those with chronic blood loss, pancreatic insufficiency, bowel disease, or Alzheimer's disease. Signs and symptoms of severe deficiency include skin changes, diarrhea, hair loss, mental disturbances, and recurrent infections. While relatively uncommon, borderline deficiency states may be seen in the elderly and are manifested by sleep and behavioral disturbances, the symptoms of inflammatory bowel disease, impaired glucose tolerance, loss of smell or taste, abnormal menstruation, impotence, infertility, reduced appetite, anorexia, and night blindness.

Food sources of zinc include oysters, shellfish, fish, red meat, pumpkin seeds, ginger root, split peas, Brazil nuts, whole wheat, rye, oats, peanuts, lima beans, almonds, potatoes, garlic, carrots, and black beans. Treatment of zinc deficiency requires 30–60 mg per day for specific needs. Most Americans consume 10 mg per day. Supplementation of 15–20 mg per day is the accepted range (Murphy, 1996).

Adverse reactions can occur with prolonged intake of 150 mg or more per day and exhibit as copper-deficiency anemia. Reduced high-density lipoprotein cholesterol levels and depressed immune function also are possible. Toxicity is rare because vomiting usually occurs if amounts large enough to be toxic are ingested. Zinc sulfate taken on an empty stomach can cause gastrointestinal upset.

Special Considerations

Zinc status can be determined by examining leukocyte zinc levels; hair and serum levels are less reliable. Zinc and copper affect absorption of one another. To promote absorption, zinc supplements should not be taken with high-fiber foods. Zinc sulfate should be taken with food. Supplementation during pregnancy is recommended. Some believe that zinc supplementation helps in the treatment of alopecia. Zinc is a component in the treatment of Wilson's disease, a rare disorder in which copper accumulates in the liver and is slowly released into the body. Because zinc interferes with copper absorption, it helps to prevent accumulation typical of Wilson's disease. No drug interactions are known (Murray, 1996).

Boron

Boron is a trace mineral that may assist in the maintenance of bone and joint function. It plays a pivotal role in calcium and magnesium metabolism.

Populations at risk for deficiency states include most Americans because the typical American diet does not include sufficient amounts of fruits and vegetables. Signs and symptoms of deficiency may include an increased risk of postmenopausal bone loss.

Food sources of boron include fruits and vegetables. Many supplement forms are available, but for wellness, sodium borate is appropriate. For the treatment of arthritis, sodium tetraborate decahydrate is recommended. The recommended dosage is 3–9 mg/day.

Adverse reactions occur with very high doses (500 mg/day) and manifest as nausea, vomiting, and diarrhea. No drug interactions are known.

Special Considerations

Individuals should be monitored for deficiency states and potential toxicities. Indications for supplementation include osteoporosis and osteoarthritis.

Summary

Nutritional therapies hold an attraction that others do not. They appear to be the most "natural" of complementary and alternative interventions. The use of nutritional supplements or special diets should not be taken lightly or undertaken without expert guidance. The potential for negative consequences always must be a consideration. However, believing that all nutritional needs can be met via whole foods is naive. In our culture, many people often are in a hurry and pressured; obtaining and properly preparing nutritional food is not a priority. Pollutants, medications, fast foods, processed foods, and existing medical conditions dictate the need for some supplementation. The choice of supplements should be specific to the individual's needs and should take into account the potential risks to the individual.

Obtaining the expert guidance of an appropriately trained and credentialed practitioner can be more complicated than one would expect. There are multiple avenues to certification: having a "certificate of attendance" is not the same as "being certified." Always be cautious when seeking expert guidance (e.g., when a practitioner proports having the "only" of something—the only substance, the only remedy, the one true supplement, the secret substance or cure). The answer(s) may not be easy to hear. True answers usually involve the patient's participation and assuming responsibility for much of what is to be accomplished. There are no magic cures.

References

Aihara, H. (1986). *Acid and alkaline.* Oroville, CA: George Ohsawa Macrobiotic Foundation.

Blackburn, G. (1997). Safe amounts of vitamins. *Health News, 3*(11), 4.

Block, G. (1991). Epidemiologic evidence regarding vitamin C and cancer. *American Journal of Clinical Nutrition, 54,* 1310S–1314S.

Block, P. (1994). *A banquet of health.* Evanston, FL: Evanston Publishing, Inc.

Bradford, M. (Ed.). (1997). *Alternative healthcare.* San Diego: Thunderbay Press.

Butterworth, C.E., Jr., Hatch, K.D., Macaluso, M., Cole, P., Sauberlich, H.E., Soong, S.J., Borst, M., & Baker, V.V. (1992) Folate deficiency and cervical dysplasia. *JAMA, 267,* 528–533.

Comstock, G.W., Alberg, A.J., Huang, H.Y., Wu, K., Burke, A.E., Hoffman, S.C., Norkus, E.P., Gross, M., Cutler, R.G., Morris, J.S., Spate, V.L., & Helzlsouer, K.J. (1997). The risk of developing lung cancer associated with antioxidants in the blood: Ascorbic acid, carotenoids, alpha-tocopherol, selenium, and total peroxyl radical absorbing capacity. *Cancer Epidemiology, Biomarkers and Prevention, 6,* 907–916.

Dagnelie, P.C., Vergote, F.J., van Staveren, W.A., van den Berg H., Dingjan, P.G., & Hautvast, J.G. (1990). High prevalence of rickets in infants on macrobiotic diets. *American Journal of Clinical Nutrition, 51,* 202–208.

Dalton, K., & Dalton, M.J. (1987). Characteristics of pyridoxine overdose neuropathy syndrome. *Acta Neurologica Scandinavica, 76,* 8–11.

A diet for epilepsy provides new hope. (1997). *Tufts University Health & Nutrition Letter, 15*(4), 6.

Garland, C.F., Comstock, G.W., Garland, F.C., Helsing, K.J., Shaw, E.K., & Gorham, E.D. (1989). Serum 25-hydroxyvitamin D and colon cancer: Eight-year prospective study. *Lancet, 2*(8673), 1176–1178.

Gershoff, S. (1996). *The Tufts University guide to total nutrition.* New York: HarperCollins.

Gerson Institute. (1996). *Gerson therapy physician's training manual 1.2.0.* Bonita, CA: Author.

Griffith, H.W. (1988). *Complete guide to vitamins, minerals and supplements.* Tucson, AZ: Fisher Books.

Guo, W., Li, J.Y., Blot, W.J., Hsing, A.W., Chen, J.S., & Fraumeni, J.F. (1990). Correlations of dietary intake and blood nutrient levels with esophageal cancer mortality in China. *Nutrition and Cancer, 13*(3), 121–127.

Hennekens, C.H., Buring, J.E., & Peto, R. (1994). Antioxidant vitamins—Benefits not yet proved. *New England Journal of Medicine, 330,* 1080–1081.

Jacobs, J. (Ed.). (1996). *The encyclopedia of alternative medicine: A complete family guide to complementary therapies.* Boston: Carlton Books Ltd.

Kaul, L., Heshmat, M.Y., Kovi, J., Jackson, M.A., Jackson, A.G. Jones, G.W., Edson, M., Enterline, J.P., Worrell, R.G., & Perry, S.L. (1987). The role of diet in prostate cancer. *Nutrition and Cancer, 9*(2–3), 123–128.

Millet, P. (1989). Nutrient intake and vitamin status of healthy vegetarians and non-vegetarians. *American Journal of Clinical Nutrition, 50,* 718–727.

Moss, R.W. (1992). *Cancer therapy: The independent consumer's guide to non-toxic treatment and prevention.* New York: Equinox Press.

Murray, M.T. (1996). Encyclopedia of nutritional supplements. Rocklin, CA: Prima Publishing.

National Cancer Institute. (1990). *Cancer facts—Unconventional methods: Gerson therapy.* Bethesda, MD: Author.

National Cancer Institute. (1992). *Cancer facts—Vitamin C.* Bethesda, MD: Author

Nursing 98 drug handbook. (1998). Springhouse, PA: Springhouse Corporation.

Parsons, T.J. (1997). Reduced bone mass in Dutch adolescents fed a macrobiotic diet in early life. *Journal of Bone and Mineral Research, 12,* 1486–1494.

Pelton, R., & Overholser, L. (1994). *Alternatives in cancer therapy.* New York: Fireside.

Preventing heart attacks: B vitamins could be the big players. (1997). *University of California at Berkeley Wellness Letter, 14*(2), 1–2.

Quillin, P., & Quillin, N. (1994). *Beating cancer with nutrition.* Tulsa: Nutrition Times Press, Inc.

Quillin, P., & Quillin, N. (1998). *Beating cancer with nutrition.* Tulsa: Nutrition Times Press, Inc.

Reed, A., James, N., & Sikora, K. (1990). Mexico: Juices, coffee enemas, and cancer. *Lancet, 336*(8716), 677–678.

Reichel, H., Koeffler, H.P., & Norman, A.W. (1989). Role of vitamin D in the endocrine system in health and disease. *New England Journal of Medicine, 320,* 980–991.

Rosenfeld, I. (1996). *Dr. Rosenfeld's guide to alternative medicine.* New York: Random House.

Simone, C.B. (1992). *Cancer and nutrition.* Garden City Park, NY: Avery Publishing Group, Inc.

Taking vitamin E to heart. (1997). *University of California at Berkeley Wellness Letter, 3*(10), 1–2.

Vitamin D toxicity may be widespread. (1997). *Tufts University Health & Nutrition Letter, 15*(8), 1.

Vitamin E and immune function. (1997). *Harvard Health Letter, 22*(9), 8.

Weil, A. (1997). *Vitamins and minerals.* New York: Ivy Books.

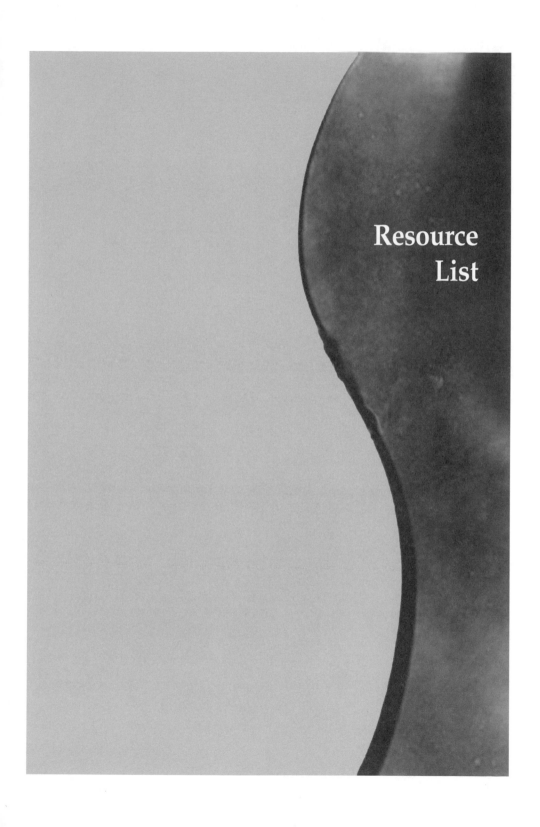

Resource
List

Resources

Alternative and Complementary Therapy Organizations

Academy of Behavioral Medicine
  Research
4301 Jones Bride Road
Bethesda, MD 20814
301-295-3270

Academy of Psychosomatic Medicine
5824 North Magnolia
Chicago, IL 60660
312-784-2025

American Academy of Environmental
  Medicine
10 East Randolph Street
New Hope, PA 18938
215-862-4544
Fax: 215-862-4583

American Academy of Neural Therapy
410 East Denny Way, Suite 18
Seattle, WA 98122
206-749-9967
Fax: 206-723-1367

American Association for Therapeutic
  Humor
222 South Meramec, Suite 303
St. Louis, MO 63105
314-863-6232
Fax: 314-863-6457

American Association of Alternative
  Healers
P.O. Box 10026
Sedona, AZ 86336-8026
530-345-8622
Web site: www.cris.com/aaah/toc.htm

American Association of Alternative
  Medicine
1000 Rutherford Road
Landrum, SC 29356
864-457-5144
Fax: 864-457-5145

American Association of
  Orthomolecular Medicine
7375 Kingsway
Burnaby, British Columbia V3N3B5
Canada

American College for Advancement in
  Medicine
231 Verdugo Drive, Suite 204
Laguna Hills, CA 92653
949-583-7666
Fax: 949-455-9679
Web site: www.acam.org

American College of Hyperbaric
  Medicine at Ocean Medical Center
4001 Ocean Drive, Suite 105
Lauderdale-by-the-Sea, FL 33308
305-771-4000

American Complementary Medical
  Association
269 Cypresswood #133
Spring, TX 77388
713-580-0705
800-680-0705
Fax: 888-729-3274

American Foundation of Traditional
  Chinese Medicine
505 Beach Street
San Francisco, CA 94133
415-776-0502
Fax: 415-776-9053

American Health Science University
1010 South Juliet Street #107
Aurora, CO 80012
303-340-2054
Fax: 303-367-2577

American Holistic Health Association
P.O. Box 17400
Anaheim, CA 92817-7400
714-779-6152
Fax: 714-777-2917
E-mail: ahha@healthy.net
Web site: www.ahha.org

American Holistic Medical Association
6728 Old McLean Village Drive
McLean, VA 22101
703-556-9245
Fax: 703-556-8729
E-mail: Holistmed@aol.com
Web site: www.holisticmedicine.org

American Holistic Nurses Association
P.O. Box 2130
Flagstaff, AZ 86003-2130
919-787-5181
800-278-2462
Fax: 919-787-4916

American Holistic Veterinary Medical
  Association
2214 Old Emmorton Road
Bel Air, MD 21015
For information, send a self-
  addressed, stamped envelope.

American Institute for Preventive
  Medicine
30445 Northwestern Highway #350
Farmington Hills, MI 48334
810-539-1808
800 345-2476
Fax: 810-649-1808

American Oriental Bodywork Therapy
  Association
1010 Haddonfield-Berlin Road, Suite 408
Voorhees, NJ 08043
609-782-1616
Fax: 609-782-1653
Web site: www.healthy.net/aobta

American Preventive Medical
  Association
9912 Georgetown Pike, Suite D2
Great Falls, VA 22066
800-230-2762
Fax: 703-759-6711
Web site: www.healthy.net

Foundation for Advancement in
  Cancer Therapy
Box 1242
Old Chelsea Station
New York, NY 10113
212-741-2790

Guild for Structural Integration
P.O. Box 1559
Boulder, CO 80306
303-447-0122
800-447-0150
Fax: 303-447-0108
Web site: www.rolfguild.org

International College of Applied
  Kinesiology
6405 Metcalf Avenue, Suite 503
Shawnee Mission, KS 66202-3929
913-542-1801
Fax: 913-542-1746

International Oxidative Medicine
  Association
P.O. Box 891954
Oklahoma City, OK 73189
405-634-1310
Fax: 405-634-7320
Web site: www.healthy.net/ioma

International Ozone Association
31 Strawberry Hill Avenue
Stamford, CT 06902
203-348-3542

International Society for
  Orthomolecular Medicine
16 Florence Avenue
Toronto, Ontario M2N 1E9
Canada
416-733-2117
Fax: 416-733-2352
E-mail: centre@orthomed.org

Acupressure

The Acupressure Institute
1533 Shattuck Avenue
Berkeley, CA 94709
510-845-1059
800-442-2232
E-mail: info@acupressure.com

American Oriental Bodywork Therapy
  Association
1010 Haddonfield-Berlin Road, Suite
  408
Voorhees, NJ 08043
609-782-1616
Fax: 609-782-1653
Web site: www.healthy.net/aobta

Acupuncture

Acupuncture Research Institute
313 West Andrix Street
Monterey Park, CA 91754
323-722-7353

American Academy of Medical
  Acupuncture
5820 Wilshire Boulevard, Suite 500
Los Angeles, CA 90036
323-937-5514
Fax: 323-937-0959
Web site: www.medicalacupuncture.com

American Acupuncture Center
2320 Woosley Street
Berkeley, CA 94705
510-843-7370

American Association of Acupuncture
  and Bio-Energetic Medicine
2512 Manoa Road
Honolulu, HI 96822
808-946-2069
Fax: 808-946-0378

American Association of Oriental
  Medicine
433 Front Street
Catasauqua, PA 18032
610-226-1433
888-500-7999
Fax: 610-264-2768
Web site: www.aaom.org

American Foundation of Traditional
  Chinese Medicine (Educator
  Programs Only)
P.O. Box 330267
San Francisco, CA 94133
415-392-7002
Fax: 415-392-7003

The Center for Integrated Medicine
3120 Southwest Freeway, Suite 41
Houston, TX 77098
713-523-4181
Fax: 713-523-4184

International Veterinary Acupuncture
  Society
2140 Conestoga Road
Chester Springs, PA 19425
Fax: 610-827-7245

Alexander Technique

Alexander Technique International
58 Shepard Street
Cambridge, MA 02138
617-876-2709

American Society for the Alexander
  Technique
401 East Market Street #17
Charlottesville, VA 22902
800-473-0620

North American Society of Teachers of
  the Alexander Technique
P.O. Box 517
Urbana, IL 61801
800-473-0620
Web site: www.alexandertech.org

Antineoplastons

Burzynski Research Institute
9432 Old Katy Road, Suite 200
Houston, TX 77055
713-335-5697

Anthroposophy

Anthroposophical Society in America
1923 Geddes Avenue
Ann Arbor, MI 48104-1797
734-930-9462
E-mail: information@anthroposophy.org
Web site: www.anthroposophy.org

Anthroposophical Therapy and
  Hygiene Association
241 Hungry Hollow Road
Chestnut Ridge, NY 10977
917-356-8499

Aromatherapy

American Alliance of Aroma Therapy
P.O. Box 309
Depoe Bay, OR 97341-0309
800-809-9850
Fax: 800-809-9808

American Aromatherapy Association
P.O. Box 3679
South Pasadena, CA 91031
818-457-1742

Aromatherapy Institute and Research
  Leydet Aromatics
P.O. Box 2354
Fair Oaks, CA 95628
916-965-7546
Fax: 916-962-3292
Web site: www.leydet.com

Aromatherapy Organizations Council
3 Latymer Close, Braybrooke
Market Harboroeigh, Leics
LE16 8LN
United Kingdom

Pacific Institute of Aromatherapy
P.O. Box 6723
San Rafael, CA 94903
415-479-9121

Art Therapy

American Art Therapy Association Inc.
1202 Allanson Road
Mundelein, IL 60060
847-949-6064
Fax: 847-566-4580
Web site: www.arttherapy.org

National Coalition of Arts Therapies
Associations
2000 Century Plaza, Suite 108
Columbia, MD 21044
410-997-4040

Ayurvedic Therapy

The American Institute of Vedic
Studies
P.O. Box 8357
Santa Fe, NM 87504
505-983-9385
Web site: www.vedanet.com

Maharishi Ayurvedic International
P.O. Box 49667
Colorado Springs, CO 80949-9667
719-260-5500
800-255-8332
Fax: 719-260-7400

Maharishi University of Management
1000 North Fourth Street
Fairfield, IA 52557
515-472-7000
Fax: 515-472-1137
Web site: www.maharishi-
medical.com or www.mum.edu

National Institute of Ayurvedic
Medicine
13 West Ninth Street
New York, NY 10011
212-505-8971
Fax: 914-278-8700
Web site: www.niam.com

Biofeedback

Association for Applied
Psychophysiology and Biofeedback
10200 West 44th Avenue, Suite 304
Wheat Ridge, CO 80033
303-422-8436
800-477-8892
Fax: 303-422-8894
Web site: www.aapb.org

Biofeedback Certification Institute of
America
10200 West 44th Avenue, Suite 304
Wheat Ridge, CO 80033
Fax: 303-422-8894
Web site: www.aapb.org

Breath Therapy

Mind/Body Medical Institute
Division of Behavioral Medicine
Beth Israel Deaconess Medical Center
110 Francis Street, Suite 1A
Boston, MA 02215
617-632-9525
Fax: 617-632-7383
Web site: http://mindbody.harvard.edu

Stress Reduction Clinic
UMASS Memorial Medical Center
Shaw Building
55 Lake Avenue North
Worcester, MA 01655
508-856-1616
Fax: 508-856-1977

Chelation Therapy

American Board of Chelation Therapy
70 West Huron Street
Chicago, IL 60610
312-266-7246

American College for Advancement in
Medicine
231 Verdugo Drive, Suite 204
Laguna Hills, CA 92653
949-583-7666
Fax: 949-455-7679

Preventive Medical Associates
13911 Ridgedale Drive
Minnetonka, MN 55305
612-593-9458

Chiropractic

American Chiropractic Association
1701 Clarendon Boulevard
Arlington, VA 22209
703-276-8800
Fax: 703-243-2593
Web site: www.amerchiro.org

International Chiropractors
Association
1110 North Glebe Road, Suite 1000
Arlington, VA 22201
703-528-5000
800-423-4690
Fax: 703-528-5023
Web site: www.chiropractic.org

National Directory of Chiropractic
P.O. Box 10056
Olathe, KS 66051
800-888-7914
Fax: 913-780-0658

World Chiropractic Alliance
2950 North Dobson Road 1
Chandler, AZ 85224
800-347-1011
Fax: 480-732-9313

Cranial Osteopathy

Cranial Academy
8202 Clearvista Parkway, 9D
Indianapolis, IN 46256
317-594-0411
Fax: 317-594-9299

Upledger Institute
11211 Prosperity Farms Road, Suite
D325
Palm Beach Gardens, FL 33410
561-622-4334
800-233-5880
Fax: 561-622-4771
Web site: www.upledger.com

Dance Therapy

American Dance Therapy Association
2000 Century Plaza, Suite 108
Columbia, MD 21044
410-997-4040
Fax: 410-997-4048
Web site: www.adta.org

Diet/Nutrition Therapies

American Academy of Nutrition
3408 Sausalito
Corona Del Mar, CA 92625-1638
714-760-5081
800-290-4226
Fax: 949-760-1788
Web site: www.nutritioneducation.com

American College of Advances in
Medicine
P.O. Box 3427
Laguna Hills, CA 92654
949-583-7666
800-532-3688
Fax: 949-455-9679
Web site: www.acam.org

American Dietetics Association
216 West Jackson Boulevard, Suite
800
Chicago, IL 60606
800-877-1600
Fax: 312-899-1979
Web site: www.eatrite.org

American Health Science University
1010 South Joliet Street #107
Aurora, CO 80012
303-340-2054
800-530-8079
Fax: 303-367-2577
Web site: www.ahsu.com

Gerson Institute
P.O. Box 430
Bonita, CA 91908
619-585-7600
888-4-GERSON
Fax: 619-585-7610
Web site: www.gerson.org

Kushi Institute of the Berkshires
P.O. Box 7
Becket, MA 01233
413-623-5742
800-975-8744
Fax: 413-623-8827
Web site: www.macrobiotics.org

National Institute of Nutritional
Education
1010 South Joliet Street #209
Aurora, CO 80012
303-340-2054
800-530-8079

Tufts University Diet and Nutrition Letter
10 High Street, Suite 706
Boston, MA 02110
617-350-7994
800-274-7581
Fax: 617-350-7974

Energetic Healing

Barbara Brennan School of Healing
P.O. Box 2005
East Hampton, NY 11937
516-329-0951
800-924-2564
Fax: 516-329-0298
Web site: www.barbarabrennan.com

Guided Imagery

Academy for Guided Imagery
P.O. Box 2070
Mill Valley, CA 94942
800-726-2070
415-389-9324
Web site: www.healthy.net/agi

Herbal Therapy

American Botanical Council
P.O. Box 144345
Austin, TX 78714-4345
512-926-4900
Fax: 512-926-2345
Web site: www.herbalgram.org

American Herbalists Guild
P.O. Box 70
Roosevelt, UT 84066
435 722-8434
Fax: 435-722-8452
Web site: www.healthy.net/herbalists

Herb Research Foundation
1007 Pearl Street, Suite 200
Boulder, CO 80303
303-449-2265
800-748-2617
Fax: 303-449-7849
Web site: www.hrf.org

Homeopathic Therapy

Foundation for Homeopathic Education
and Research
2124 Kittredge Street
Berkeley, CA 94704
510-649-8930
Fax: 510-649-1955

Homeopathic Academy of
Naturopathic Physicians
12132 SE Foster Place
Portland, OR 97266
513-761-3298
Fax: 503-762-1929
Web site: www.healthy.net/hanp

Homeopathic Educational Services
2124 Kittredge Street
Berkeley, CA 94704
510-649-0294
Fax: 510-649-1955
Web site: www.homeopathic.com

The National Center for Homeopathy
801 North Fairfax Street, Suite 306
Alexandria, VA 22314
703-548-7790
Fax: 703-548-7792
Web site: www.homeopathic.org

Horticultural Therapy

American Horticultural Therapy
Association
909 York Street
Denver, CO 80206
303-820-3151
Fax: 303-820-3844
Web site: www.ahta.org

Hypnosis/Hypnotherapy

Academy of Scientific Hypnotherapy
P.O. Box 12041
San Diego, CA 92112
619-427-6225
Fax: 619-427-5650

American Board of Hypnotherapy
16842 Von Karman Avenue #475
Irvine, CA 92714
800-872-9996
Fax: 949-251-4632

American Council of Hypnotist
Examiners
700 South Central Avenue
Glendale, CA 91204
818-242-5378
Fax: 818-247-9379

The American Society of Clinical
Hypnosis
33 West Grand
Chicago, IL 60610
312-645-9810
Fax: 312-645-9818

International Medical and Dental
Hypnotherapy Association
4110 Edgeland, Suite 800
Royal Oaks, MI 48073-2251
800-257-5467
Fax: 248-549-5421

National Guild of Hypnotists
P.O. Box 308
Merrimack, NH 03054
603-429-9438
Fax: 603-424-8066

Massage Therapy
American CranioSacral Therapy
Association
11211 Prosperity Farms Road, D-325
Palm Beach Gardens, FL 33410-3487
800-311-9204
E-mail: acsta@iahe.com

American Massage Therapy Association
820 Davis Street, Suite 100
Evanston, IL 60201-4444
847-864-0123
Web site: www.amtamassage.org

American Reike Master Association
P.O. Box 130
Lake City, FL 32056
904-755-9638
Fax: 904-755-9638

Associated Bodyworks and Massage
Professionals
28677 Buffalo Park Road
Evergreen, CO 80439-7347
800-458-2267
303-674-8479
Fax: 303-674-0859
Web site: www.abmp.com

The Feldenkrais Guild of North America
3611 SW Hood, Suite 100
Portland, OR 97201
503-221-6612
Fax: 503-221-6618
Web site: www.feldenkrais.com

Hellerwork International
The Body of Knowledge
406 Berry Street
Mt. Shasta, CA 96067
530-926-2500
Fax: 530-926-6839
Web site: www.hellerwork.com

The Reiki Alliance
P.O. Box 41
Catalado, ID 83810
208-783-3535
Fax: 208-783-4848

Trager Institute
21 Locust Avenue
Mill Valley, CA 94941
415-388-2688
Fax: 415-388-2710
Web site: www.trager.com

Meditation and Stress Management
Himalayan International Institute of
Yoga Science and Philosophy
Center for Health and Healing
RR 1, Box 400
Honesdale, PA 18431-9706
570-253-5551
Fax: 570-253-9078
E-mail: chh@himalayaninstitute.org
Web site:
www.himalayaninstuitute.org

Insight Meditation Society
1230 Pleasant Street
Barre, MA 01005
978-355-4378
Fax: 978-355-6398
Web site: www.dharma.org

Institute of Noetic Sciences
P.O. Box 909
Sausalito, CA 94966
415-331-5650
Fax: 415-331-5673
Web site: www.noetic.org

Institute of Transpersonal Psychology
744 San Antonio Road
Palo Alto, CA 94303
650-493-4430
Fax: 650-493-6835
E-mail: itpinfo@itp.edu
Web site: www.itp.edu

Maharishi Ayur-Ved Products
International, Inc.
1068 Elkton Drive
Colorado Springs, CO 88107
800-255-8332
Fax: 719-260-7400
Web site: www.mapi.com

Maharishi University of Management
1000 North Fourth Street
Fairfield, IA 52557
515-472-7000
Fax: 515-472-1137
Web site: www.maharishi-
medical.com or www.mum.edu

Mind/Body Medical Institute and
Division of Behavioral Medicine
110 Francis Street, Suite 1A
Boston, MA 02215
617-632-9530
Fax: 617-632-7383

Mind/Body Health Sciences Inc.
Joan Borysenko, PhD
393 Dixon Road
Boulder, CO 80302
303-440-8460
Write for newsletter.

Stress Reduction Clinic
University of Massachusetts Medical
Center
55 Lake Avenue North
Worcester, MA 01655
508-856-1616

Music Therapy
The American Music Therapy
Association
8455 Colesville Road, Suite 1000
Silver Spring, MD 20910
301-589-3300
Fax: 301-589-5175
Web site: www.musictherapy.org

The Chalice of Repose Project
312 East Pine Street
Missoula, MT 59802
406-542-0001, ext. 2810
Fax: 406-329-5614

Guided Imagery and Music Therapy
Temple University
Presser Hall, Room 129
2001 North 13th Street
Philadelphia, PA 19122
215-204-8301

Life Sounding the Soul
Emma K. O'Brien, BMUS, RMT
The Royal Melbourne Hospital
Grattan Street
Parkville, Victoria 3050
Australia
011-613-9342-8410
Fax: 011-613-9341-7508

Sound, Listening and Learning Center
2701 East Camelback, Suite 205
Phoenix, AZ 85016
602-381-0086
Fax: 602-957-6741
Web site: www.soundlistening.com

Native American Health Care

American Indian Heritage Foundation
6051 Arlington Boulevard
Falls Church, VA 22044
202-INDIANS
Web site: www.indians.org

Native American Student Affairs Office
University of Arizona
1642 East Helen Street
Tucson, AZ
520-621-3835

The National Indian Health Board
1385 South Colorado Boulevard, Suite
A-707
Denver, CO 80222
303-759-3075
Fax: 303-759-3674
Web site: www.nihb.org

The National Native American AIDS
Prevention Center
134 Linden Street
Oakland, CA 94607
510-444-2051
Fax: 510-444-1593
Web site: www.nnaapc.org

Naturopathy

American Association of Naturopathic
Physicians
601 Valley Street, Suite 105
Seattle, WA 98109
206-298-0125
Fax: 206-298-0129
E-mail: aanp@usa.net
Web site: www.anma.net

Osteopathy

American Academy of Osteopathy
3500 DePauw Boulevard, Suite 1080
Indianapolis, IN 46268
317-879-1881
Fax: 317-879-0563

American Osteopathic Association
143 East Ontario Street
Chicago, IL 60611-2864
312-280-5800
800-621-1773

Past Life Therapy

The Association for Past Life Research
and Therapies
P.O. Box 20151
Riverside, CA 92516-0151
909-784-1570
Fax: 909-784-1570
Web site: www.arpt.com

The Society for Advancement of Past
Life Research and Therapy
774 Princcton Place
Rockville, MD 20850
301-738-2297
Fax: 301-699-0693

Pet Therapy

American Pet Association
P.O. Box 18869
Boulder, CO 80308
303-403-9222
800-272-7387
Web site: www.apapets.com

The Delta Society
289 Perimeter Road East
Renton, WA 98055-1329
800-869-6898
Fax: 541-341-5927

Therapy Dogs International
88 Bartley Road
Flanders, NJ 07836
973-252-9800
Fax: 973-252-7171
Web site: www.tdi-dog.org

Poetry Therapy

National Association for Poetry
Therapy
225 Williams Street
Huron, OH 44839
416-433-5018

Polarity Therapy

American Polarity Therapy
Association
P.O. Box 19858
Boulder, CO 80308
303-545-2080
Fax: 303-545-2161
Web site: www.polaritytherapy.org

Heartwood Institute
220 Harmony Lane
Garberville, CA 95542
Fax: 707-923-5010

Psychotherapy

American Counseling Association
5999 Stevenson Avenue
Alexandria, VA 22304-9800
703-823-9800

American Psychological Association
750 First Street NE
Washington, DC 20002
800-964-2000

American Society of Group
Psychotherapy and Psychodrama
c/o Ed Garcia
301 North Harrison Street, Suite 508
Princeton, NJ 08540
609-452-1339
Fax: 609-936-1659

Association for Applied
Psychophysiology and Biofeedback
10200 West 44th Avenue #304
Wheat Ridge, CO 80033-2840
303-422-8436
800-477-8892
Fax: 303-422-8894

Qigong

American Association of Oriental
  Medicine
433 Front Street
Catasauqua, PA 18032
610-226-1433
888-500-7999
Fax: 610-264-2768
Web site: www.aaom.org

American Foundation of Traditional
  Chinese Medicine
P.O. Box 330267
San Francisco, CA 94133
415-392-7002
Fax: 415-392-7003

East-West Academy of Healing Arts
  Qigong Institute
450 Sutter Street, Suite 2104
San Francisco, CA 94108
415-788-2227
Fax: 415-788-2242

Reflexology

American Reflexology Certification
  Board
P.O. Box 620607
Littleton, CO 80162
303-933-6921

Foot Reflexology Awareness Association
P.O. Box 7622
Mission Hills, CA 91346
818-361-0528
Fax: 818-361-0538

International Institute of Reflexology
5650 First Avenue North
P.O. Box 12642
St. Petersburg, FL 33733-2642
727-343-4811
Fax: 727-381-2807

Reflexology Association of America
4012 Rainbow Boulevard
Box K-PHB 585
Las Vegas, NV 89103-2055
702-871-9522

Reflexology Research
P.O. Box 35820, Station D
Albuquerque, NM 87176
505-344-9392
Fax: 505-344-0246

Relaxation

Mind/Body Medical Institute
Division of Behavioral Medicine
Beth Israel Deaconess Medical Center
110 Francis Street, Suite 1A
Boston, MA 02215
617-632-9525
Fax: 617-632-7383
Web site: http://mindbody.harvard.edu/

Rolfing

The Rolf Institute
205 Canyon Boulevard
Boulder, CO 80302
800-530-8875
Fax: 303-449-5978
Web site: www.rolf.org

Shamanism

Dance of the Deer Foundation for the
  Study of Huichol Shamanism
P.O. Box 699
Soquel, CA 95703
831-475-9560
Web site: www.shamanism.com

The Foundation for Shamanic Studies
P.O. Box 1939
Mill Valley, CA 94942
415-380-8282
Fax: 415-380-8416

Shiatsu

The School for Oriental Medicine
The New Center for Wholistic Health
  Education and Research Team
6801 Jericho Turnpike
Syosset, NY 11791-4413
516-364-0808
Fax: 516-364-0989

Tai Chi

Look under "Martial Arts" in the
  yellow pages for classes in your
  area.

Therapeutic Touch

Nurse Healers-Professional Associates
1211 Locust Street
Philadelphia, PA 19107

215-545-8079
Fax: 215-545-8107
E-mail: nhpa@nursecominc.com
Web site: www.therapeutic-touch.org

Traditional Oriental Medicine

See Acupressure, Acupuncture

Yoga

American Yoga Association
P.O. Box 19986
Sarasota, FL 34236
941-927-4977
Fax: 941-921-9844

Ayurvedic Institute
11311 Menaud NE, Suite A
Albuquerque, NM 87112
505-291-9698
Fax: 505-294-7572
Web site: www.ayurvedic.com

College of Maharishi Ayurvedic
  Medicine Health Center
1603 North Fourth Street
Fairfield, IA 52557
515-472-8477
Fax: 515-472-7379
Web site: www.mum.edu

Integral Yoga Institute
227 West 13th Street
New York, NY 10011
212-929-0585
Fax: 212-675-3674

Samata Yoga and Health Institute
4150 Tivoli Avenue
Los Angeles, CA 90066
310-306-8845
Fax: 310-306-4632
Web site: www.samata.com

Yoga Research & Education Center
P.O. Box 1386
Lower Lake, CA 95457
707-928-9898
Fax: 707-928-4738

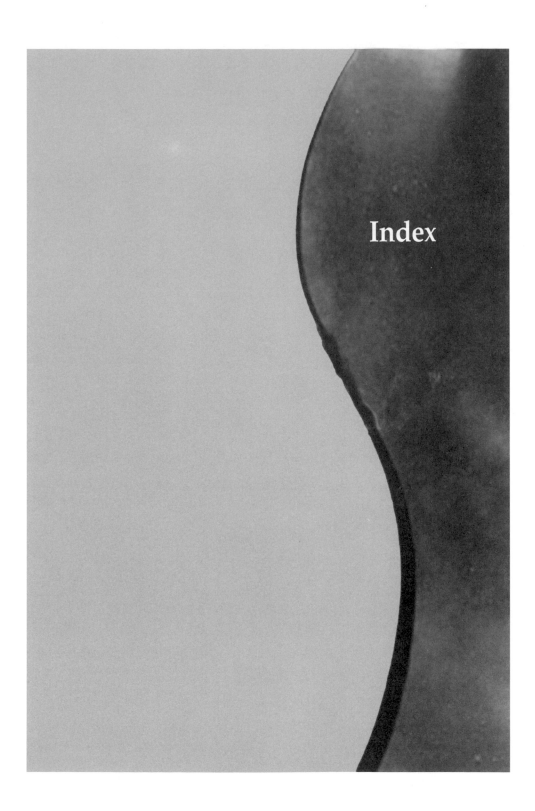

Index

Index

The letter f after a page number indicates a figure or figures; the letter t indicates a table.